CHEMO DIET COOKBOOK FOR THE NEWLY DIAGNOSED

Essential Recipes and Guidance to Support You During and After Cancer Treatment

Kingsley Klopp

Copyright © 2024 All rights reserved.

No part of this book may be reproduced or transmitted in any form or by any means, electronic or mechanical, including photocopying, recording, or by any information storage and retrieval system, without written permission from the author. The scanning, uploading, and distribution of this book via the internet or via any other means without the permission of the author is illegal and punishable by law. The author has made every effort to ensure the accuracy of the information contained in this book. However, the author cannot be held responsible for any errors or omissions.

Table of Contents

Part 1: Understanding Chemotherapy and Nutrition
- What is Chemotherapy?..9
- Common Side Effects..11
- Why Nutrition Matters..14
- Key Nutrients for Cancer Patients...16
- Foods to Stock Up On for Pre-Chemotherapy Preparation..........................18
- Managing Appetite Changes..21
- Coping with Nausea and Vomiting During Chemotherapy..........................24
- Foods to Avoid During Chemotherapy..26

Breakfast Recipes
Lentil and Veggie Breakfast Salad..30
Savory Porridge with Egg..31
Granola and Fruit Medley..32
Savory Muffins..33
Protein-Packed French Toast...34
Spinach and Cheese Stuffed Mushrooms...35
Veggie-Packed Breakfast Burritos...36
Baked Sweet Potato with Yogurt...37
Sweet Corn Porridge..38
Overnight Barley...39
Gluten-Free Blueberry Waffles..40
Almond Butter Banana Smoothie..41
Tofu Scramble with Avocado..42
Cream of Wheat with Fruit..43
Mashed Potato Pancakes..44
Zucchini Bread...45
Turkey and Spinach Mini Quiches...46
Pumpkin Pancakes...47
Berry Yogurt Parfait..48
Banana Almond Muffins..49

Fish & Seafood Recipes
Ginger Salmon Stir-Fry...50
Baked Cod with Lemon and Dill...51
Shrimp and Avocado Salad..52

Simple Grilled Tilapia..53
Oven-Roasted Trout with Thyme...54
Pesto Shrimp Pasta..55
Clam Soup with Vegetables...56
Crab and Spinach Stuffed Mushrooms..57
Mild White Fish Soup..58
Salmon and Rice Casserole...59
Steamed Scallops with Ginger..60
Poached Haddock in Milk...61
Baked Tilapia with Oats Crust..62
Crab Salad with Light Mayo...63
 Mackerel Pate..64
Grilled Salmon with Mango Salsa..65
Sea Bass with Roasted Vegetables..66
Shrimp and Spinach Quiche...67
Parmesan Crusted Halibut..68
Tuna Steak with Tomato Salsa..69
Fish Fillet with Light Dill Sauce...70

Poultry Recipes
Ginger Chicken Congee...71
Lemon Herb Roasted Chicken..72
Turkey Sweet Potato Skillet...73
Garlic Thyme Chicken Soup...74
Baked Turkey Meatballs with Spinach..75
Chicken Stew with Soft Vegetables..76
Turkey and Zucchini Burgers...77
Simple Poached Chicken...78
Creamy Chicken and Mushroom Soup...79
Soft Chicken Tacos with Guacamole...80
Turkey Sloppy Joes...81
Chicken Porridge with Mild Spices...82
Pesto Chicken Pasta with Whole Wheat Noodles..................................83
Chicken and Broccoli Alfredo...84
Turkey Breast with Sweet Potato Mash...85
Slow-Cooked Chicken with Root Vegetables...86
Chicken Salad with Greek Yogurt Dressing...87
Turkey Quinoa Stuffed Peppers...88
Chicken Ginger Noodle Soup..89
Moroccan Spiced Chicken Stew...90
Chicken Paillard with Steamed Greens...91

Soup & Stew Recipes

Beet and Cabbage Red Soup..92
Moroccan Lentil Soup..93
Asparagus Soup...94
Kale and White Bean Soup..95
Mulligatawny Soup..96
French Onion Soup..97
Spiced Pumpkin and Carrot Stew..98
Potato Leek Soup...99
Corn Chowder..100
Cabbage Soup..101
Cauliflower and Leek Soup..102
Oxtail Stew..103
Zucchini Basil Soup...104
 Italian Wedding Soup...105
Broccoli and Cheese Soup...106
Vegetable Beef Soup..107
Split Pea and Ham Soup..108
Thai Coconut Chicken Soup..109
Lentil and Carrot Soup..110
Spinach and Potato Stew...111

Vegetables

Steamed Broccoli with Lemon Zest...112
Carrot and Zucchini Ribbons..113
Roasted Beetroot with Feta...114
 Sautéed Green Beans with Almonds...115
Cauliflower Steaks...116
 Herb Roasted Parsnips..117
Grilled Asparagus with Lemon Butter...118
Sweet Potato Casserole...119
Braised Red Cabbage..120
Eggplant Parmesan..121
Roasted Brussels Sprouts with Garlic...122
Bok Choy with Oyster Sauce...123
Corn on the Cob with Herb Butter..124
Cucumber Salad with Dill...125
Spaghetti Squash with Tomato Sauce...126
Roasted Garlic Mashed Potatoes..127
Pea and Mint Puree...128
Roasted Turnips with Rosemary...129
Swiss Chard with Pine Nuts..130
Fennel and Orange Salad..131

10-WEEK MEAL PLAN..132

Important Note

Welcome to the **Chemo Diet Cookbook for the Newly Diagnosed**. We're thrilled to have you join us on this journey towards finding nourishment and comfort through thoughtfully crafted recipes designed to support you during chemotherapy. As you explore the pages of this cookbook, we hope you discover new flavors, rediscover the joy of eating, and feel empowered in your culinary endeavors.

However, it's essential to remember that each person's journey with cancer and chemotherapy is unique, and so are their dietary needs. While our recipes are created with care and consideration for common chemotherapy side effects, they might not perfectly align with your individual requirements. Your body is unique, and what works for one person may not work for another.

Adjusting to Your Needs: We encourage you to use this cookbook as a flexible guide. Feel free to tweak and modify the recipes to suit your personal tastes and nutritional needs. Whether it's adjusting the seasoning to better match your taste preferences or substituting ingredients based on your tolerance and availability, make these recipes your own.

Consult Your Healthcare Team: If you ever feel uncertain about a particular ingredient or recipe, please consult with your healthcare team. Your doctors, nutritionists, and dietitians know your medical history and current condition best, and their guidance is invaluable. They can provide personalized advice to ensure that the food you're eating supports your health and treatment plan optimally.

Additionally, while we've provided nutritional information for each recipe, please understand that these values are approximate. The nutritional content can vary based on factors such as ingredient brands, portion sizes, and preparation methods. We recommend using this information as a general guide and adjusting as needed to meet your specific dietary requirements.

Furthermore, If our cookbook has brought joy to your kitchen and table, we'd be thrilled to hear about your experiences in an Amazon review. On the flip side, if you stumble upon any hiccups while exploring our recipes, don't hesitate to get in touch at **kloppkingsley@gmail.com**. We're here to support your cooking journey every step of the way.

To show our appreciation for your purchase, we're delighted to offer you these special bonuses as a heartfelt thank you.

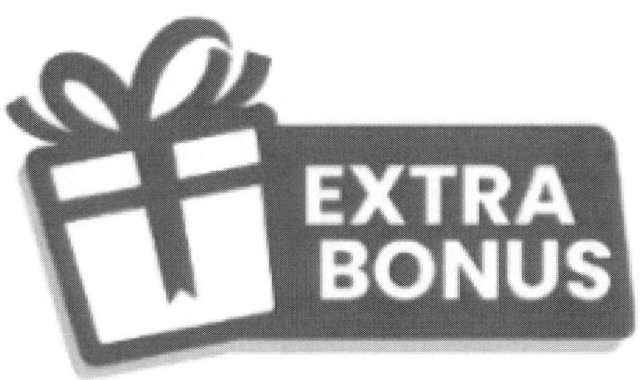

1. A Food Tracker Journal
2. Downloadable E-BOOK featuring full-color images of finished recipes

Introduction

Imagine this: you've just left the doctor's office with a diagnosis that's turned your world upside down. You're now part of a club you never wanted to join—the club of cancer patients. The word "chemo" looms large, a daunting specter that seems to overshadow everything, especially the simple joy of eating. But what if I told you that the journey you're about to embark on doesn't have to be as overwhelming as it seems? What if I told you that there's a way to turn the necessity of a chemo-friendly diet into a celebration of flavor, health, and resilience? Welcome to the **Chemo Diet Cookbook for the Newly Diagnose**d, a lifeline for navigating the culinary challenges that lie ahead with confidence and creativity. Cancer treatment, particularly chemotherapy, can feel like an endless uphill battle. The side effects are numerous and varied, ranging from nausea and fatigue to changes in taste and appetite. It's enough to make anyone feel like food is their enemy. But here's the good news: food can be your ally. This cookbook is designed to transform your kitchen into a sanctuary of healing, providing you with the tools and recipes to nourish your body and soul during this challenging time.

Let's face it: the internet is flooded with generic advice about what to eat during chemotherapy. But the "Chemo Diet Cookbook for the Newly Diagnosed" is different. This is not just a collection of recipes; it's a comprehensive guide that speaks directly to you—the newly diagnosed. Each recipe has been crafted with care, considering not just nutritional value, but also the practicalities of preparation and the likelihood of appealing to a chemo-altered palate. We understand that when you're dealing with the side effects of treatment, the last thing you need is complicated cooking instructions or hard-to-find ingredients. Simplicity, ease, and flavor are at the heart of every dish in this book. Let's talk about taste for a moment. Chemotherapy can wreak havoc on your taste buds, making your favorite foods taste metallic, bland, or just plain weird. It's frustrating, to say the least. This cookbook is packed with tips and tricks to enhance flavor, making food enjoyable again. From zesty marinades to aromatic herbs, we'll show you how to coax the best out of every ingredient, ensuring that your meals are not just nutritious, but also delicious.

In addition to recipes, we've included practical advice on meal planning, shopping, and prepping. We understand that energy levels can vary greatly during treatment, so we've provided strategies for making the most of your good days and managing the tough ones. Batch cooking, freezer-friendly meals, and quick, nutritious snacks all feature prominently, ensuring that you're never left wondering what to eat when you're too tired to cook.

And let's not forget the importance of variety. The monotony of eating the same bland foods day in and day out can be dispiriting. This cookbook offers a wide range of recipes, from comforting soups and stews to vibrant salads and smoothies, all designed to cater to different cravings and nutritional needs. Whether you're looking for a hearty breakfast to start your day, a light lunch to keep you going, or a satisfying dinner to end on a positive note, we've got you covered.

As you set out on this new chapter, remember that every meal is an opportunity to support your body and uplift your spirit. The "Chemo Diet Cookbook for the Newly Diagnosed" is here to help you do just that. Let's turn the challenge of a chemo diet into an adventure of discovery and nourishment, one delicious bite at a time.

Part 1: Understanding Chemotherapy and Nutrition

What is Chemotherapy?

Chemotherapy is a term that evokes a complex blend of emotions, especially for those embarking on the daunting journey of cancer treatment. It refers to a type of cancer treatment that uses drugs to destroy cancer cells, preventing them from growing and dividing. The essence of chemotherapy lies in its goal: to eliminate cancer cells with precision while trying to minimize harm to the body's healthy cells. It is a battle within the body, a fight for survival, strength, and hope.

The story of chemotherapy is one of scientific curiosity, relentless pursuit, and human resilience. The journey began in the early 20th century, during the grim days of World War II. Researchers observed that soldiers exposed to mustard gas experienced significantly lowered white blood cell counts. This observation led to the hypothesis that such compounds could be used to target rapidly dividing cancer cells. By the 1940s, the first chemotherapy agent, nitrogen mustard, was being tested and showed promise in treating lymphoma, marking the beginning of a new era in cancer treatment. As the decades passed, the field of chemotherapy evolved, driven by scientific breakthroughs and an unwavering commitment to improve patient outcomes. The 1950s and 60s saw the discovery of several key chemotherapeutic agents, including methotrexate, which led to the first cures of metastatic cancer and acute leukemia in children. These milestones were monumental, offering a glimmer of hope to patients and families devastated by cancer diagnoses. The 1970s and 80s heralded a period of refinement and expansion. Researchers developed combination chemotherapy regimens, using multiple drugs to target cancer cells in different ways. This approach not only improved efficacy but also reduced the likelihood of resistance, where cancer cells adapt to evade treatment. These advancements transformed chemotherapy from a rudimentary, often toxic intervention into a more sophisticated and effective therapy.

Today, chemotherapy continues to be a cornerstone of cancer treatment, often used in conjunction with surgery, radiation, and newer targeted therapies. Modern chemotherapy is more nuanced, tailored to the specific type of cancer, its stage, and the individual patient's health and needs. This personalization has enhanced the effectiveness of treatment while striving to reduce side effects, making the journey a little less arduous. Despite these advances, the emotional toll of chemotherapy is profound. The mere mention of the word can stir feelings of fear, anxiety, and uncertainty. Patients often grapple with the anticipation of side effects, the disruption to their daily lives, and the psychological burden of battling a life-threatening illness. Yet, within this struggle lies an incredible reservoir of human spirit and resilience.

Patients undergoing chemotherapy often describe their journey in terms of courage and determination. Each treatment session is a step forward, a testament to their strength and will to fight. Support from family, friends, and healthcare providers forms an essential pillar, providing comfort and encouragement when it is needed most. The shared stories of survivors inspire hope, reminding those in the midst of treatment that they are not alone and that victory over cancer is possible. The history of chemotherapy is a testament to the power of scientific innovation and human perseverance. From its origins in wartime observations to its current role as a tailored, precise treatment modality, chemotherapy has transformed the landscape of cancer care. It is not merely a medical intervention but a symbol of hope and progress in the fight against cancer.

As we look to the future, the ongoing research and development in cancer treatment continue to hold promise. Advances in understanding the genetic and molecular underpinnings of cancer are paving the way for even more targeted and effective therapies. The journey of chemotherapy is far from over, and with each step forward, we move closer to a world where cancer can be managed, treated, and ultimately conquered.

Common Side Effects of Chemotherapy

Chemotherapy, while a powerful weapon in the fight against cancer, often comes with a range of side effects that can significantly impact a patient's quality of life. Understanding these side effects is crucial for preparing mentally and physically for the journey ahead. It's important to remember that everyone's experience with chemotherapy is unique, and side effects can vary in type and intensity from person to person.

1. Fatigue
One of the most pervasive side effects of chemotherapy is fatigue. This is not just ordinary tiredness but a profound sense of exhaustion that doesn't improve with rest. Fatigue can be caused by the treatment itself, the cancer, or a combination of both. It can make even simple daily activities feel overwhelming and can persist long after treatment has ended.

2. Nausea and Vomiting
Chemotherapy drugs can irritate the stomach lining and affect the brain's area that controls nausea and vomiting. These side effects can be immediate or delayed, sometimes occurring hours or days after treatment. Fortunately, advances in anti-nausea medications have made it possible to manage these symptoms more effectively than in the past.

3. Hair Loss (Alopecia)
Hair loss is one of the most visible and emotionally challenging side effects of chemotherapy. Chemotherapy targets rapidly dividing cells, which includes cancer cells as well as hair follicles. Hair loss can occur all over the body, including the scalp, eyebrows, and eyelashes. The extent and duration of hair loss depend on the type and dosage of chemotherapy drugs used.

4. Mouth Sores (Mucositis)
Chemotherapy can damage the cells lining the mouth and digestive tract, leading to painful sores and ulcers. This condition, known as mucositis, can make eating and drinking difficult and increase the risk of infection. Good oral hygiene and specific mouthwashes can help manage this side effect.

5. Loss of Appetite
Many patients experience a loss of appetite during chemotherapy, which can be due to nausea, taste changes, or the psychological stress of treatment. This can lead to weight loss and nutritional deficiencies, making it important to focus on nutrient-rich foods and sometimes seek guidance from a nutritionist.

6. Changes in Taste and Smell
Chemotherapy can alter the sense of taste and smell, making food taste metallic, bland, or otherwise unappetizing. These changes can be frustrating and can contribute to the loss of appetite. Experimenting with different flavors and textures may help make food more palatable.

7. Skin and Nail Changes
Skin may become dry, itchy, or red, and some patients develop a rash. Nails can become brittle, discolored, or develop ridges. It's essential to protect the skin from the sun and avoid harsh chemicals that can exacerbate these symptoms.

8. Anemia
Chemotherapy can reduce the bone marrow's ability to produce red blood cells, leading to anemia. Symptoms of anemia include fatigue, shortness of breath, and dizziness. Blood transfusions or medications to boost red blood cell production may be necessary in severe cases.

9. Increased Risk of Infections
Since chemotherapy affects the bone marrow's production of white blood cells, the body's ability to fight infections is compromised. Patients are more susceptible to infections and must take precautions such as avoiding large crowds and practicing good hygiene.

10. Bleeding and Bruising
A lower platelet count, another result of chemotherapy's impact on bone marrow, can lead to easy bruising and bleeding. Patients may notice frequent nosebleeds, bleeding gums, or prolonged bleeding from cuts. Being gentle and avoiding activities that could cause injury is crucial.

11. Cognitive Changes (Chemo Brain)
Some patients experience cognitive changes, often referred to as "chemo brain," which include difficulties with memory, concentration, and multi-tasking. These changes can be subtle or more pronounced and usually improve over time after treatment ends.

12. Emotional and Psychological Effects
The emotional toll of chemotherapy cannot be understated. Anxiety, depression, and emotional distress are common as patients navigate the physical and psychological challenges of treatment. Support from loved ones, counseling, and support groups can be invaluable during this time.

Coping with Side Effects
Managing the side effects of chemotherapy requires a multifaceted approach. Here are some strategies that can help:
- Medication: There are many medications available to manage specific side effects, such as anti-nausea drugs, pain relievers, and growth factors for blood cells.
- Nutrition: Maintaining a balanced diet and staying hydrated can help mitigate some side effects and support overall health.

- Rest: Allowing for plenty of rest and pacing activities can help manage fatigue.
- Support: Emotional and psychological support from family, friends, and professional counselors can provide comfort and resilience.
- Communication: Regular communication with the healthcare team is essential to address side effects promptly and adjust treatment plans as necessary.

Why Nutrition Matters

When facing the battle against cancer, nutrition becomes a vital ally in the journey. The role of nutrition in chemotherapy is profoundly significant, offering more than just sustenance; it becomes a cornerstone of strength, resilience, and healing. For patients undergoing chemotherapy, good nutrition can make a world of difference in their treatment experience and overall well-being.

The Foundation of Strength and Healing
Chemotherapy is a powerful treatment designed to target and destroy cancer cells. However, it also takes a toll on healthy cells and the body's overall energy reserves. Proper nutrition provides the essential fuel needed to support the body's ability to repair itself and maintain strength during this grueling process. When your body is nourished, it can better withstand the side effects of treatment, enhance your immune response, and improve your quality of life.

Imagine your body as a fortress under siege; nutrition is the reinforcements that strengthen your defenses, repair the walls, and keep your soldiers (your immune cells) ready for the next battle. Without adequate nutrition, this fortress weakens, making it harder to fight the enemy.

Enhancing Treatment Efficacy
The effectiveness of chemotherapy can be influenced by a patient's nutritional status. Well-nourished bodies are better equipped to handle the full course of treatment without interruption. Conversely, malnutrition can lead to treatment delays or dose reductions, potentially compromising the therapy's effectiveness. Maintaining a balanced diet helps ensure that your body can tolerate and respond optimally to the treatment.

Managing Side Effects
Chemotherapy often brings a host of side effects, such as nausea, vomiting, mouth sores, and taste changes. These can make eating a challenge and lead to poor nutritional intake. Thoughtful nutrition planning can help mitigate these side effects. For instance, consuming small, frequent meals can help manage nausea, while soft, easy-to-swallow foods can be more palatable for those with mouth sores. Imagine being in a turbulent sea; proper nutrition acts like a lifeboat, providing stability and support amidst the waves of side effects. It can make the difference between feeling overwhelmed and finding a sense of control and comfort.

Supporting Immune Function
Chemotherapy can weaken the immune system, making it more difficult to fend off infections. Nutrient-rich foods bolster the immune system, helping to maintain its ability to protect the body. Vitamins, minerals, antioxidants, and proteins play critical roles in supporting immune function and healing processes.

Picture your immune system as an army that relies on a steady supply of resources. Good nutrition ensures that this army is well-equipped to fight off any threats that may arise, keeping you safer and more resilient.

Emotional and Psychological Well-being

Food is not just fuel; it's also a source of comfort and pleasure. During chemotherapy, maintaining a connection to the enjoyment of eating can be a significant emotional boost. Preparing and sharing meals with loved ones can provide a sense of normalcy and joy amidst the upheaval of treatment.

The act of nourishing yourself is an act of self-love and empowerment. It's a reminder that even in the face of adversity, you are taking active steps to care for your body and soul.

Practical Tips for Nutritional Support

To optimize your nutrition during chemotherapy, consider these practical tips:

1. Eat Small, Frequent Meals: This can help manage nausea and keep energy levels stable.
2. Stay Hydrated: Drinking plenty of fluids is crucial to prevent dehydration, especially if experiencing vomiting or diarrhea.
3. Focus on Protein: Protein is essential for repairing body tissues and maintaining muscle mass. Include lean meats, eggs, dairy, beans, and nuts in your diet.
4. Incorporate Fruits and Vegetables: These are rich in vitamins, minerals, and antioxidants that support your immune system and overall health.
5. Listen to Your Body: Eat when you're hungry and don't force yourself if you're not. Adjust your eating habits to what feels best for you.
6. Seek Professional Guidance: A registered dietitian specializing in oncology can provide personalized nutrition advice tailored to your specific needs and treatment plan.

Key Nutrients for Cancer Patients

1. Protein
Importance: Protein is vital for the repair and regeneration of tissues, maintaining muscle mass, and supporting the immune system. During cancer treatment, the body's protein needs increase due to the stress of the illness and the impact of treatments.
Sources: Lean meats (chicken, turkey), fish, eggs, dairy products (milk, cheese, yogurt), legumes (beans, lentils), nuts, seeds, and soy products (tofu, tempeh).
Tips: Include a source of protein in every meal and snack. For those experiencing appetite loss or difficulty eating, protein shakes or supplements can be helpful.

2. Carbohydrates
Importance: Carbohydrates provide the primary source of energy for the body. They are essential for maintaining energy levels, especially when undergoing the physically taxing processes of cancer treatment.
Sources: Whole grains (brown rice, quinoa, oats), fruits, vegetables, legumes, and starchy vegetables (sweet potatoes, corn).
Tips: Choose complex carbohydrates over simple sugars to provide sustained energy and additional nutrients. Aim to include a variety of colorful fruits and vegetables to maximize nutrient intake.

3. Fats
Importance: Healthy fats are crucial for brain function, hormone production, and absorption of fat-soluble vitamins (A, D, E, K). They also provide a concentrated source of energy.
Sources: Avocados, nuts, seeds, olive oil, flaxseed oil, fatty fish (salmon, mackerel, sardines), and nut butters.
Tips: Incorporate sources of healthy fats into meals and snacks. Avoid trans fats and limit saturated fats, focusing instead on monounsaturated and polyunsaturated fats.

4. Vitamins and Minerals
Importance: Vitamins and minerals are essential for numerous bodily functions, including immune support, energy production, and cellular repair.

Key Vitamins:
- Vitamin C: Boosts the immune system and helps in the repair of tissues. Sources: Citrus fruits, strawberries, bell peppers, and broccoli.
- Vitamin D: Important for bone health and immune function. Sources: Sunlight exposure, fortified dairy products, fatty fish, and supplements if necessary.
- Vitamin E: Acts as an antioxidant, protecting cells from damage. Sources: Nuts, seeds, spinach, and broccoli.
- Folate (Vitamin B9): Crucial for DNA repair and synthesis. Sources: Leafy green vegetables, legumes, and fortified cereals.
- Vitamin B12: Important for nerve function and blood cell production. Sources: Meat, fish, dairy, and fortified plant-based products.

Key Minerals:
- Iron: Necessary for oxygen transport in the blood. Sources: Red meat, poultry, fish, legumes, and fortified cereals.
- Calcium: Essential for bone health. Sources: Dairy products, leafy greens, and fortified plant-based milks.
- Magnesium: Involved in muscle and nerve function, energy production. Sources: Nuts, seeds, whole grains, and leafy greens.
- Zinc: Supports the immune system and aids in wound healing. Sources: Meat, shellfish, legumes, and seeds.

Tips: Aim for a balanced diet that includes a variety of foods to ensure adequate intake of these essential vitamins and minerals. Supplements may be necessary if dietary intake is insufficient or if recommended by a healthcare provider.

5. Antioxidants

Importance: Antioxidants help protect the body's cells from damage caused by free radicals. They play a role in reducing inflammation and supporting the immune system.

Sources: Berries (blueberries, strawberries, raspberries), dark leafy greens (kale, spinach), nuts, seeds, green tea, and colorful vegetables (carrots, bell peppers).

Tips: Incorporate a rainbow of fruits and vegetables into your diet to maximize antioxidant intake. Be mindful of high-dose antioxidant supplements, as they may interact with cancer treatments.

6. Fiber

Importance: Fiber supports digestive health, helps maintain regular bowel movements, and can aid in controlling blood sugar levels.

Sources: Whole grains, fruits, vegetables, legumes, nuts, and seeds.

Tips: Gradually increase fiber intake and ensure adequate hydration to prevent digestive discomfort. Include a mix of soluble and insoluble fiber for comprehensive digestive health benefits.

7. Water

Importance: Hydration is crucial for all bodily functions, including nutrient transport, temperature regulation, and waste elimination. Cancer treatments can increase the risk of dehydration.

Sources: Water, herbal teas, broths, and water-rich fruits and vegetables (cucumbers, watermelon, oranges).

Tips: Aim to drink at least 8-10 glasses of water per day, adjusting for individual needs and treatment-related fluid losses. Carry a water bottle and sip throughout the day to maintain hydration.

Foods to Stock Up On for Pre-Chemotherapy Preparation

1. Lean Proteins
Importance: Protein is crucial for maintaining muscle mass, repairing tissues, and supporting the immune system during chemotherapy.
Foods to Stock Up On:
- Chicken and Turkey: Skinless, boneless cuts can be quickly cooked and added to various dishes.
- Fish: Salmon, mackerel, and other fatty fish are excellent sources of protein and omega-3 fatty acids, which help reduce inflammation.
- Eggs: Versatile and easy to prepare, eggs provide a high-quality protein source.
- Legumes: Beans, lentils, and chickpeas are great plant-based protein options.
- Tofu and Tempeh: These soy products are excellent for vegetarians and can be used in a variety of dishes.

Tips: Cook and freeze portions of lean meats and fish for quick meals. Keep canned beans and legumes on hand for easy additions to soups, salads, and stews.

2. Whole Grains
Importance: Whole grains provide sustained energy and are rich in fiber, which helps with digestion and maintaining steady blood sugar levels.
Foods to Stock Up On:
- Oats: Ideal for quick breakfasts or snacks.
- Brown Rice and Quinoa: These grains can be cooked in batches and used in various dishes.
- Whole Wheat Pasta: A healthier alternative to regular pasta, providing more fiber and nutrients.
- Barley and Farro: Nutritious grains that can be added to soups and salads.
- Whole Grain Bread: Opt for bread with minimal added sugars and preservatives.

Tips: Cook large batches of grains and freeze them in portion-sized containers for convenience.

3. Fruits and Vegetables
Importance: Fruits and vegetables are rich in vitamins, minerals, and antioxidants, which help support the immune system and overall health.
Foods to Stock Up On:
- Berries: Blueberries, strawberries, and raspberries are high in antioxidants and can be frozen for smoothies or snacks.
- Leafy Greens: Spinach, kale, and Swiss chard are packed with nutrients and can be used in salads, soups, and smoothies.
- Cruciferous Vegetables: Broccoli, cauliflower, and Brussels sprouts are known for their cancer-fighting properties.

- Root Vegetables: Carrots, sweet potatoes, and beets provide essential vitamins and minerals.
- Citrus Fruits: Oranges, lemons, and grapefruits are high in vitamin C, which supports the immune system.

Tips: Buy fresh fruits and vegetables in season, and freeze them for later use. Pre-wash and cut vegetables for easy snacking and meal prep.

4. Dairy and Dairy Alternatives

Importance: Dairy products and their alternatives provide essential nutrients like calcium, vitamin D, and protein.

Foods to Stock Up On:
- Milk and Plant-Based Milks: Almond, soy, and oat milk are great alternatives for those who are lactose intolerant.
- Yogurt: Greek yogurt is particularly high in protein and can be a soothing snack.
- Cheese: Opt for low-fat varieties and use them to add flavor to meals.
- Cottage Cheese: A versatile and high-protein option.

Tips: Choose plain yogurt to avoid added sugars, and add fresh fruit or honey for sweetness.

5. Healthy Fats

Importance: Healthy fats are essential for brain health, hormone production, and the absorption of fat-soluble vitamins.

Foods to Stock Up On:
- Avocados: High in healthy fats and versatile in various dishes.
- Nuts and Seeds: Almonds, walnuts, chia seeds, and flaxseeds are great for snacking or adding to meals.
- Olive Oil: Use for cooking or as a dressing for salads.
- Nut Butters: Peanut butter, almond butter, and other nut butters are convenient sources of healthy fats and protein.

Tips: Store nuts and seeds in the refrigerator to keep them fresh longer.

6. Hydration Essentials

Importance: Staying hydrated is crucial during chemotherapy to help manage side effects like nausea, constipation, and fatigue.

Foods and Drinks to Stock Up On:
- Water: Keep plenty of bottled or filtered water on hand.
- Herbal Teas: Ginger, peppermint, and chamomile teas can help soothe nausea and provide hydration.
- Electrolyte Drinks: Look for low-sugar options to help maintain electrolyte balance.
- Broths and Soups: Chicken broth, vegetable broth, and miso soup can be hydrating and soothing.

Tips: Infuse water with fruits and herbs for added flavor, and keep a variety of herbal teas available to suit your preferences.

7. Comfort Foods and Easy-to-Digest Options

Importance: During chemotherapy, your appetite and digestive system may be sensitive, so having easy-to-digest and comforting foods is important.

Foods to Stock Up On:
- Crackers and Toast: Plain, whole grain options are gentle on the stomach.
- Applesauce and Canned Fruit: Look for unsweetened varieties.
- Pudding and Gelatin: These can be soothing and easy to eat.
- Mashed Potatoes: A comforting and easy-to-digest option.

Tips: Keep these foods on hand for days when eating feels particularly challenging.

Managing Appetite Changes

Chemotherapy can significantly impact your appetite, making it difficult to maintain proper nutrition at a time when your body needs it most. These appetite changes can manifest as a loss of appetite, changes in taste and smell, nausea, or even increased appetite. Managing these changes is crucial for ensuring that you get the nutrients you need to support your body through treatment and recovery.

1. Understanding Appetite Changes
Importance: Understanding the reasons behind appetite changes can help you better address them.
Tips:
- Treatment Side Effects: Chemotherapy can cause nausea, vomiting, and changes in taste and smell, all of which can reduce your desire to eat.
- Emotional Factors: Stress, anxiety, and depression, common during cancer treatment, can also affect your appetite.
- Physical Changes: Chemotherapy can alter the way your body digests and absorbs food, leading to a lack of interest in eating.

2. Eating Small, Frequent Meals
Importance: Eating smaller meals more frequently can help ensure you're getting enough nutrients without overwhelming your digestive system.
Tips:
- Meal Schedule: Aim to eat five to six small meals or snacks throughout the day rather than three large meals.
- Easy-to-Eat Foods: Choose foods that are easy to prepare and eat, such as yogurt, smoothies, and soups.
- Set Reminders: Use alarms or reminders to prompt you to eat at regular intervals, especially if you're not feeling hungry.

3. Making Food More Appealing
Importance: Enhancing the appeal of food can help stimulate your appetite and make eating more enjoyable.
Tips:
- Variety and Color: Incorporate a variety of colors and textures into your meals to make them more visually appealing.
- Seasoning and Herbs: Use herbs, spices, and seasonings to add flavor to your food, especially if your taste has changed.
- Temperature: Experiment with different temperatures; some people find cold foods more palatable, while others prefer warm meals.

4. Managing Taste and Smell Changes
Importance: Changes in taste and smell can make certain foods unappealing or even repulsive.

Tips:
- Avoid Strong Smells: If strong odors bother you, opt for cold or room-temperature foods, which tend to have milder aromas.
- Masking Bitter Tastes: Use sweet or tart flavors, such as citrus or berries, to mask bitter or metallic tastes.
- Rinse Your Mouth: Rinse your mouth with a mild saltwater solution before meals to help reduce unpleasant tastes.

5. Coping with Nausea

Importance: Nausea is a common side effect of chemotherapy that can severely impact your ability to eat.

Tips:
- Ginger: Incorporate ginger into your diet through ginger tea, ginger ale, or ginger chews, as it can help reduce nausea.
- Dry Foods: Eat dry, bland foods like crackers, toast, and pretzels, especially in the morning or if you're feeling queasy.
- Stay Hydrated: Sip on clear fluids like water, broth, or herbal tea throughout the day to stay hydrated without filling up too much.

6. Boosting Calorie and Nutrient Intake

Importance: If you're eating less, it's crucial to make every bite count by focusing on nutrient-dense and calorie-rich foods.

Tips:
- Add Healthy Fats: Incorporate healthy fats like avocados, nuts, seeds, and olive oil into your meals to increase calorie intake.
- Protein-Rich Foods: Include protein sources such as eggs, dairy, lean meats, and legumes in your diet to support muscle maintenance and repair.
- Fortified Foods: Use fortified foods and supplements, such as protein powders or meal replacement shakes, to boost nutrient intake.

7. Hydration is Key

Importance: Staying hydrated is essential for overall health and can help manage some side effects of chemotherapy.

Tips:
- Drink Regularly: Aim to drink fluids regularly throughout the day, even if you're not feeling thirsty.
- Variety of Beverages: Include a variety of hydrating beverages such as water, herbal teas, clear broths, and diluted fruit juices.
- Monitor Intake: Keep track of your fluid intake to ensure you're meeting your hydration needs.

8. Emotional and Psychological Support

Importance: Emotional well-being is closely linked to appetite, and addressing psychological factors can help improve your desire to eat.

Tips:
- Support Groups: Join support groups where you can share experiences and gain encouragement from others undergoing similar treatments.
- Counseling: Consider speaking with a counselor or therapist who specializes in cancer care to help manage stress and anxiety.
- Mindful Eating: Practice mindful eating techniques to enhance your connection with food and enjoy meals more fully.

Coping with Nausea and Vomiting During Chemotherapy

Nausea and vomiting are among the most distressing side effects of chemotherapy, affecting many patients during their treatment journey. These symptoms can significantly impact your quality of life, appetite, and overall well-being. However, there are effective strategies and treatments available to help manage and alleviate these symptoms.

Understanding the Causes
Importance: Knowing why nausea and vomiting occur can help you better manage these symptoms.
Tips:
- Chemotherapy Drugs: Certain chemotherapy drugs are more likely to cause nausea and vomiting. Discuss with your doctor which medications might affect you and the expected severity.
- Gastrointestinal Tract and Brain Interaction: Chemotherapy can irritate the lining of the stomach and intestines, and it can also trigger the brain's vomiting center.
- Other Factors: Anxiety, motion, certain smells, and even the anticipation of treatment can contribute to nausea.

Medications to Manage Nausea
Importance: Anti-nausea medications, also known as antiemetics, are crucial in controlling these symptoms.
Tips:
- Prescribed Antiemetics: Your oncologist can prescribe medications such as ondansetron (Zofran), metoclopramide (Reglan), or dexamethasone to prevent and treat nausea and vomiting.
- Take as Directed: Follow the prescribed schedule for antiemetics, even if you feel fine, to prevent nausea before it starts.
- Communicate with Your Doctor: If your current medication isn't effective, inform your healthcare provider. There are multiple antiemetics, and finding the right one or combination may take time.

Dietary Adjustments
Importance: What you eat and drink can have a significant impact on managing nausea.
Tips:
- Small, Frequent Meals: Eating small amounts throughout the day can prevent an empty stomach, which can exacerbate nausea.
- Bland Foods: Opt for bland, easy-to-digest foods like crackers, toast, bananas, rice, and applesauce.

- Cold or Room-Temperature Foods: These can be less aromatic and more tolerable than hot foods, which can have stronger smells that trigger nausea.
- Avoid Greasy, Spicy, or Fried Foods: These can be harder to digest and may worsen nausea.
- Hydration: Sip on clear liquids like water, broth, herbal teas, or electrolyte drinks throughout the day to stay hydrated. Avoid caffeinated and carbonated beverages, which can irritate the stomach.
- Ginger and Peppermint: Ginger in various forms (tea, ginger ale, ginger chews) and peppermint tea can help soothe the stomach.

Behavioral and Environmental Strategies

Importance: Making changes to your environment and daily habits can help manage nausea.

Tips:
- Rest After Eating: Sit upright or recline with your head elevated for about an hour after eating to help digestion.
- Fresh Air: Ensure good ventilation in your home. Fresh air can help reduce feelings of nausea.
- Avoid Strong Smells: Stay away from cooking smells, perfumes, smoke, and other strong odors that can trigger nausea.
- Wear Loose Clothing: Tight clothing around the waist can increase discomfort and nausea.
- Relaxation Techniques: Practice deep breathing, meditation, or guided imagery to reduce anxiety and stress, which can exacerbate nausea.

Alternative and Complementary Therapies

Importance: Some patients find relief through alternative therapies, which can be used alongside conventional treatments.

Tips:
- Acupuncture: Some studies suggest that acupuncture can help reduce chemotherapy-induced nausea and vomiting.
- Aromatherapy: Essential oils like lavender, peppermint, and ginger can be soothing. Inhale directly from the bottle or use a diffuser.
- Acupressure: Applying pressure to specific points on the body, such as the wrist (P6 point), can help alleviate nausea.

Support and Counseling

Importance: Emotional and psychological support is crucial when dealing with persistent nausea and vomiting.

Tips:
- Counseling and Support Groups: Talking to a counselor or joining a support group can help you manage the emotional aspects of nausea and vomiting.
- Stress Reduction: Activities like yoga, gentle exercise, and hobbies can help distract you from nausea and improve overall well-being.
- Education: Learning more about your treatment and its side effects can reduce anxiety and help you feel more in control.

Foods to Avoid During Chemotherapy

1. Raw or Undercooked Foods

Importance: Chemotherapy can weaken the immune system, making it harder for your body to fight off infections. Raw or undercooked foods can harbor harmful bacteria and increase the risk of foodborne illnesses.

Foods to Avoid:
- Raw Meat and Poultry: Avoid sushi, steak tartare, and any other dishes that include raw or undercooked meat or poultry.
- Raw Fish and Shellfish: Steer clear of sushi, sashimi, raw oysters, clams, and other uncooked seafood.
- Unpasteurized Dairy Products: Skip unpasteurized milk, cheese, and yogurt, as they can contain harmful bacteria.
- Undercooked Eggs: Avoid foods made with raw or undercooked eggs, such as homemade mayonnaise, Caesar salad dressing, and certain desserts like mousse or tiramisu.

Tips: Ensure all meat, poultry, fish, and eggs are cooked thoroughly to safe internal temperatures. Use a food thermometer to check for doneness.

2. Foods High in Added Sugars

Importance: While it's important to maintain energy levels during chemotherapy, foods high in added sugars can lead to energy spikes and crashes, contribute to weight gain, and may weaken the immune system.

Foods to Avoid:
- Sugary Beverages: Soda, energy drinks, sweetened teas, and fruit punches.
- Sweets and Desserts: Candy, cookies, cakes, pastries, and ice cream with high sugar content.
- Processed Snacks: Packaged snacks like granola bars, cereals, and flavored yogurt often contain added sugars.

Tips: Opt for naturally sweetened foods like fruits and choose whole, unprocessed snacks. Read labels to identify and avoid products with added sugars.

3. Fried and Greasy Foods

Importance: Fried and greasy foods can be difficult to digest and may worsen nausea, vomiting, and other gastrointestinal issues common during chemotherapy.

Foods to Avoid:
- Fried Fast Food: Fried chicken, French fries, onion rings, and other fried fast food items.
- Greasy Snacks: Potato chips, nachos, and other greasy snacks.
- Heavy Sauces and Gravies: Foods drenched in heavy, greasy sauces or gravies.

Tips: Choose baked, grilled, or steamed options instead of fried foods. Prepare meals with healthy fats like olive oil or avocado.

4. Spicy Foods

Importance: Spicy foods can irritate the digestive tract, leading to discomfort, heartburn, and exacerbated mouth sores, which are common side effects of chemotherapy.

Foods to Avoid:
- Hot Peppers: Jalapeños, habaneros, and other hot peppers.
- Spicy Sauces and Seasonings: Hot sauce, chili powder, and other spicy condiments.
- Spicy Prepared Meals: Spicy curries, tacos, and other dishes with a high level of spiciness.

Tips: Use mild seasonings and herbs to flavor your food instead. If you enjoy some heat, opt for milder options like bell peppers or a small amount of mild salsa.

5. High-Fiber Foods

Importance: While fiber is important for digestive health, high-fiber foods can sometimes cause bloating, gas, and discomfort, especially if you're experiencing digestive issues from chemotherapy.

Foods to Avoid:
- Raw Vegetables: Especially cruciferous vegetables like broccoli, cauliflower, and Brussels sprouts.
- Whole Grains: Foods like bran cereals, whole grain bread, and brown rice.
- Legumes: Beans, lentils, and chickpeas can be hard to digest.

Tips: Opt for cooked vegetables, refined grains like white rice and pasta, and peel fruits to reduce fiber content. Introduce fiber slowly back into your diet as tolerated.

6. Acidic Foods

Importance: Acidic foods can irritate the mouth and throat, particularly if you have mouth sores, a common side effect of chemotherapy.

Foods to Avoid:
- Citrus Fruits: Oranges, lemons, grapefruits, and other citrus fruits.
- Tomato Products: Tomato sauce, ketchup, and other tomato-based products.
- Vinegar-Based Foods: Pickles, vinaigrette dressings, and other vinegar-based foods.

Tips: Choose non-acidic fruits like bananas, melons, and applesauce. Use alternatives to tomato-based sauces, such as cream or cheese sauces.

7. Dairy Products (For Some)

Importance: Some people undergoing chemotherapy may develop lactose intolerance or find that dairy products exacerbate nausea and digestive issues.

Foods to Avoid:
- Milk: Whole, skim, and flavored milk.
- Cheese: Particularly soft cheeses which may be harder to digest.
- Ice Cream: Regular ice cream can be high in lactose and sugar.

Tips: Try lactose-free dairy products or plant-based alternatives like almond milk, soy milk, and dairy-free yogurt. Hard cheeses and yogurt with live cultures might be easier to digest.

8. Alcohol

Importance: Alcohol can irritate the digestive system, interact with chemotherapy drugs, and exacerbate dehydration and other side effects.

Tips: Avoid alcohol during chemotherapy treatment. Opt for non-alcoholic beverages like sparkling water with a splash of juice, herbal teas, or mocktails.

9. Caffeinated Beverages

Importance: Caffeine can lead to dehydration and increase anxiety and insomnia, which can be problematic during chemotherapy.

Foods to Avoid:
- Coffee: Regular and decaffeinated coffee if it irritates your stomach.
- Energy Drinks: These often contain high levels of caffeine and sugar.
- Certain Teas and Sodas: Check labels for caffeine content.

Tips: Drink plenty of water, herbal teas, and other non-caffeinated beverages. Decaffeinated versions of your favorite drinks might be a good alternative.

Further Clarification

We cannot emphasize this enough: the impact of chemotherapy on individuals can vary greatly. What works harmoniously for one person may induce unexpected reactions in another. As such, it's crucial to recognize that the recipes featured in this cookbook are crafted specifically for those undergoing or who have undergone chemotherapy. Each individual's body responds uniquely to treatments and dietary adjustments. Chemotherapy can alter taste preferences, digestion, and overall tolerance to certain foods. While we have curated these recipes with care and consideration, we urge you to remain attentive to your body's signals. If you find that a particular ingredient triggers discomfort or intolerance, we encourage you to substitute or adjust it accordingly. Furthermore, consulting with your healthcare team—comprising oncologists, dietitians, and other specialists—is vital. They can provide personalized advice tailored to your specific medical needs and treatment plan. Your health and well-being are our utmost priority, and we want your experience with this cookbook to be both supportive and empowering. It's also important to note that the nutritional information provided alongside each recipe is intended as a general guideline. Variations in ingredients, portion sizes, and preparation methods can affect nutritional values. Therefore, we recommend using this information as a reference point while adapting recipes to suit your dietary requirements.

Above all, we understand the emotional and physical challenges that come with chemotherapy. Our goal is to offer not only nourishing meal options but also a sense of comfort and reassurance during this time. We hope that the "**Chemo Diet Cookbook for the Newly Diagnosed**" serves as a valuable resource in your journey towards wellness.

Breakfast Recipes

1. Lentil and Veggie Breakfast Salad
Ingredients:
- 1 cup cooked lentils
- 1 cup cherry tomatoes, halved
- 1 small cucumber, diced
- 1/2 red bell pepper, diced
- 1/4 cup red onion, finely chopped
- 1 avocado, diced
- 1/4 cup fresh parsley, chopped
- 2 tbsp olive oil
- 1 tbsp lemon juice
- 1 tsp cumin
- 1/2 tsp paprika
- 1/4 tsp black pepper

Instructions:
1. In a large bowl, combine the cooked lentils, cherry tomatoes, cucumber, red bell pepper, red onion, avocado, and parsley.
2. In a small bowl, whisk together the olive oil, lemon juice, cumin, paprika, and black pepper.
3. Pour the dressing over the salad and toss gently to combine.
4. Serve immediately or refrigerate until ready to eat.

Nutrition Info (per serving):
- Calories: 250
- Protein: 9g
- Carbohydrates: 23g
- Dietary Fiber: 9g
- Sugars: 5g
- Fat: 15g
- Saturated Fat: 2g
- Cholesterol: 0mg
- Sodium: 25mg

Servings: 2
Cooking Time: 15 minutes

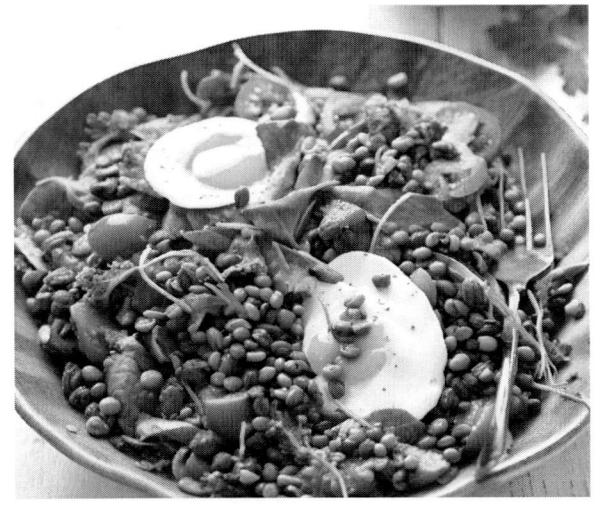

2. Savory Porridge with Egg

Ingredients:
- 1/2 cup rolled oats
- 1 cup water
- 1/2 cup low-sodium vegetable broth
- 1/4 cup shredded carrots
- 1/4 cup chopped spinach
- 1 egg
- 1/2 tsp turmeric
- 1/4 tsp black pepper
- 1 tbsp chopped fresh chives

Instructions:
1. In a saucepan, bring the water and vegetable broth to a boil. Add the oats, shredded carrots, and turmeric. Reduce heat to low and simmer for 5 minutes, stirring occasionally.
2. Stir in the chopped spinach and continue to cook for another 2-3 minutes until the oats are tender and the spinach is wilted.
3. In a small nonstick skillet, cook the egg sunny-side up or to your preference.
4. Pour the porridge into a bowl and top with the cooked egg.
5. Sprinkle with black pepper and fresh chives before serving.

Nutrition Info (per serving):
- Calories: 230
- Protein: 10g
- Carbohydrates: 28g
- Dietary Fiber: 5g
- Sugars: 3g
- Fat: 8g
- Saturated Fat: 2g
- Cholesterol: 185mg
- Sodium: 100mg

Servings: 1
Cooking Time: 15 minutes

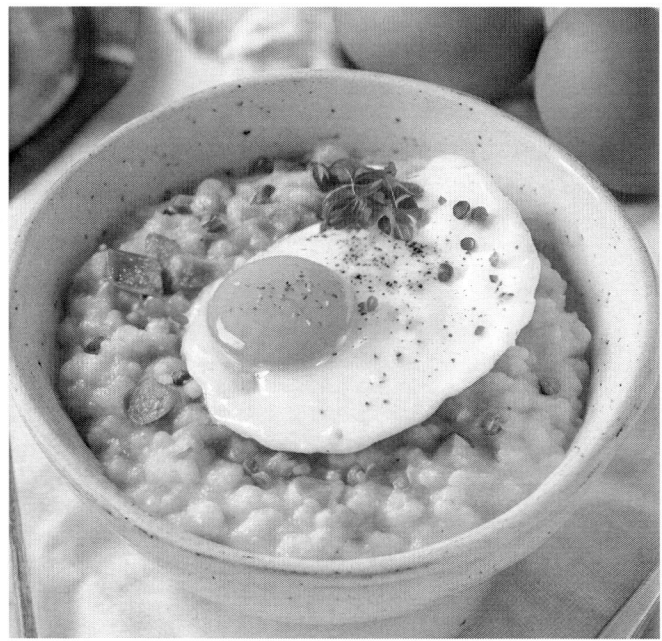

3. Granola and Fruit Medley

Ingredients:
- 1 cup rolled oats
- 1/4 cup chopped almonds
- 1/4 cup pumpkin seeds
- 1/4 cup dried cranberries
- 1/4 cup honey
- 2 tbsp coconut oil
- 1 tsp vanilla extract
- 1/2 cup Greek yogurt
- 1/2 cup mixed berries (blueberries, strawberries, raspberries)
- 1 small banana, sliced

Instructions:
1. Preheat your oven to 325°F (165°C). In a large bowl, combine the oats, almonds, pumpkin seeds, and dried cranberries.
2. In a small saucepan, heat the honey and coconut oil over low heat until melted. Remove from heat and stir in the vanilla extract.
3. Pour the honey mixture over the oat mixture and stir until well combined.
4. Spread the mixture onto a baking sheet lined with parchment paper and bake for 15-20 minutes, stirring halfway through, until golden brown. Let cool completely.
5. In serving bowls, layer the Greek yogurt, granola, and mixed berries. Top with banana slices before serving.

Nutrition Info (per serving):
- Calories: 300
- Protein: 7g
- Carbohydrates: 45g
- Dietary Fiber: 5g
- Sugars: 25g
- Fat: 12g
- Saturated Fat: 6g
- Cholesterol: 0mg
- Sodium: 20mg

Servings: 2
Cooking Time: 30 minutes

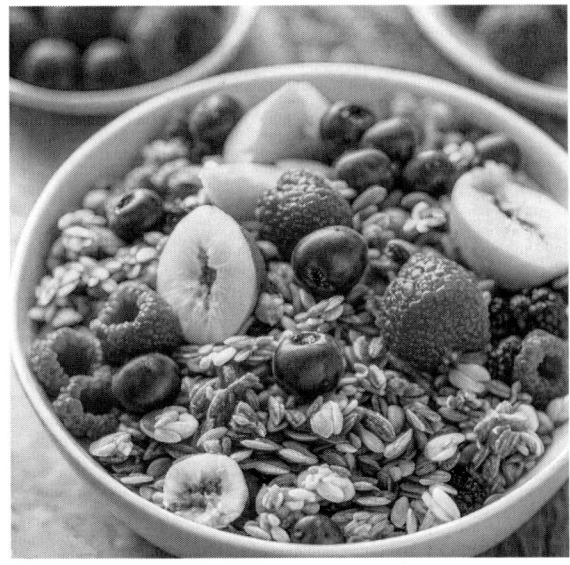

4. Savory Muffins

Ingredients:
- 1 cup whole wheat flour
- 1/2 cup rolled oats
- 1 tsp baking powder
- 1/2 tsp baking soda
- 1/2 tsp black pepper
- 1/2 tsp garlic powder
- 1/4 cup grated Parmesan cheese
- 1/2 cup grated zucchini, squeezed dry
- 1/2 cup grated carrot
- 1/4 cup chopped fresh parsley
- 2 eggs
- 1/2 cup low-fat milk
- 1/4 cup olive oil

Instructions:
1. Preheat your oven to 350°F (175°C) and line a muffin tin with paper liners.
2. In a large bowl, whisk together the flour, oats, baking powder, baking soda, black pepper, garlic powder, and Parmesan cheese.
3. Add the grated zucchini, carrot, and parsley to the dry ingredients and mix well.
4. In a separate bowl, whisk together the eggs, milk, and olive oil.
5. Pour the wet ingredients into the dry ingredients and stir until just combined.
6. Divide the batter evenly among the muffin cups.
7. Bake for 20-25 minutes, or until a toothpick inserted into the center of a muffin comes out clean. Let cool on a wire rack before serving.

Nutrition Info (per serving):
- Calories: 180
- Protein: 5g
- Carbohydrates: 20g
- Dietary Fiber: 3g
- Sugars: 2g
- Fat: 9g
- Saturated Fat: 2g
- Cholesterol: 45mg
- Sodium: 160mg

Servings: 12 muffins
Cooking Time: 35 minutes

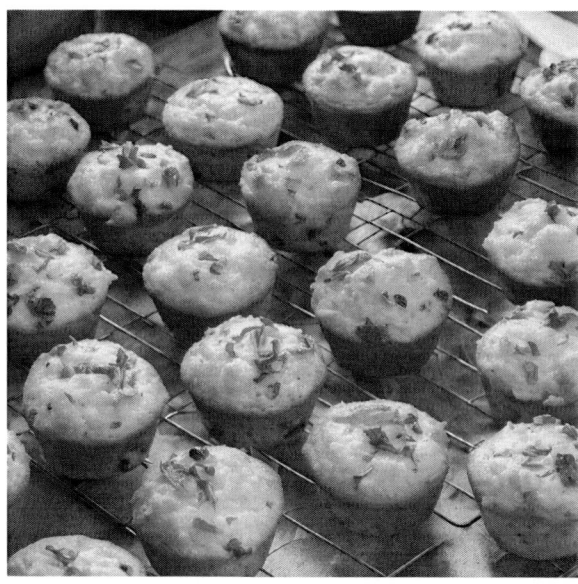

5. Protein-Packed French Toast

Ingredients:
- 4 slices whole grain bread
- 4 eggs
- 1/2 cup low-fat milk
- 1 tsp vanilla extract
- 1 tsp cinnamon
- 1 tbsp coconut oil or olive oil for cooking
- 1/4 cup Greek yogurt
- 1/2 cup fresh berries (blueberries, strawberries, raspberries)
- 1 tbsp honey or maple syrup

Instructions:
1. In a bowl, whisk together the eggs, milk, vanilla extract, and cinnamon until well combined.
2. Heat the coconut oil or olive oil in a large non-stick skillet over medium heat.
3. Dip each slice of bread into the egg mixture, ensuring both sides are well-coated.
4. Place the soaked bread slices onto the skillet and cook until golden brown on each side, about 2-3 minutes per side.
5. Serve the French toast topped with Greek yogurt, fresh berries, and a drizzle of honey or maple syrup.

Nutrition Info (per serving):
- Calories: 320
- Protein: 15g
- Carbohydrates: 42g
- Dietary Fiber: 6g
- Sugars: 12g
- Fat: 10g
- Saturated Fat: 3g
- Cholesterol: 210mg
- Sodium: 280mg

Servings: 2
Cooking Time: 20 minutes

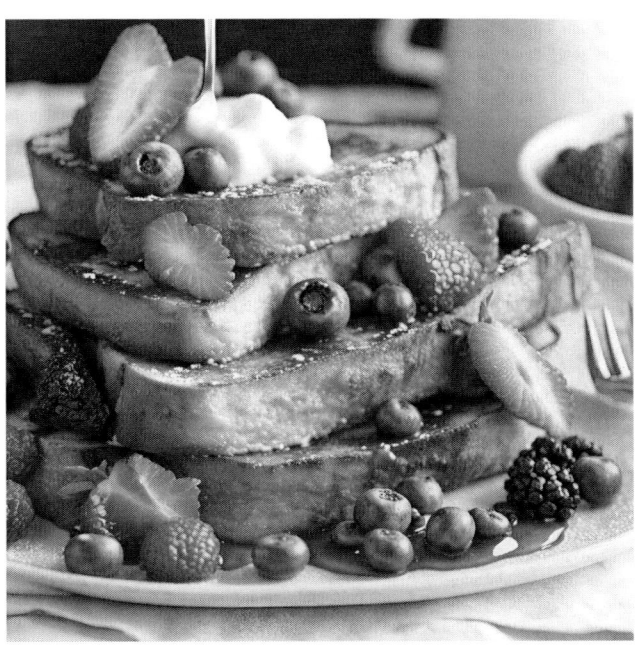

6. Spinach and Cheese Stuffed Mushrooms

Ingredients:
- 8 large portobello mushrooms, stems removed and cleaned
- 2 cups fresh spinach, chopped
- 1/2 cup ricotta cheese
- 1/2 cup shredded mozzarella cheese
- 1/4 cup grated Parmesan cheese
- 1 tsp garlic powder
- 1/4 tsp black pepper
- 1 tbsp olive oil

Instructions:
1. Preheat the oven to 375°F (190°C). Line a baking sheet with parchment paper.
2. In a skillet, heat the olive oil over medium heat. Add the chopped spinach and cook until wilted, about 3-4 minutes.
3. In a bowl, mix together the cooked spinach, ricotta cheese, mozzarella cheese, Parmesan cheese, garlic powder, and black pepper.
4. Spoon the cheese and spinach mixture into the mushroom caps, distributing evenly.
5. Place the stuffed mushrooms on the baking sheet and bake for 20 minutes, or until the mushrooms are tender and the cheese is melted and golden.
6. Serve warm.

Nutrition Info (per serving):
- Calories: 140
- Protein: 10g
- Carbohydrates: 6g
- Dietary Fiber: 2g
- Sugars: 2g
- Fat: 9g
- Saturated Fat: 4g
- Cholesterol: 25mg
- Sodium: 180mg

Servings: 4
Cooking Time: 30 minutes

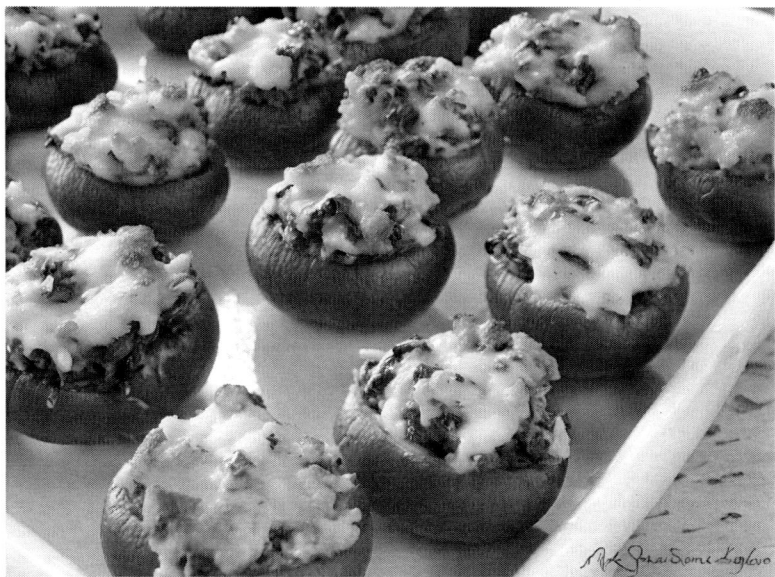

7. Veggie-Packed Breakfast Burritos

Ingredients:
- 4 whole wheat tortillas
- 1 cup black beans, drained and rinsed
- 1 cup diced bell peppers (red, green, yellow)
- 1/2 cup diced onions
- 1 cup baby spinach
- 4 eggs
- 1/2 cup shredded cheddar cheese
- 1 tbsp olive oil
- 1/4 tsp paprika
- 1/4 tsp cumin

Instructions:
1. In a large skillet, heat the olive oil over medium heat. Add the diced onions and bell peppers and cook until softened, about 5 minutes.
2. Add the black beans, baby spinach, paprika, and cumin to the skillet. Cook until the spinach is wilted and everything is heated through, about 3 minutes.
3. In a separate pan, scramble the eggs until cooked through.
4. Warm the tortillas in the microwave or on a skillet until pliable.
5. Assemble the burritos by placing the veggie mixture and scrambled eggs in the center of each tortilla. Sprinkle with cheddar cheese.
6. Fold the sides of the tortilla over the filling, then roll it up tightly.
7. Serve immediately or wrap in foil and refrigerate for later.

Nutrition Info (per serving):
- Calories: 320
- Protein: 18g
- Carbohydrates: 38g
- Dietary Fiber: 8g
- Sugars: 4g
- Fat: 12g
- Saturated Fat: 4g
- Cholesterol: 185mg
- Sodium: 350mg

Servings: 4
Cooking Time: 20 minutes

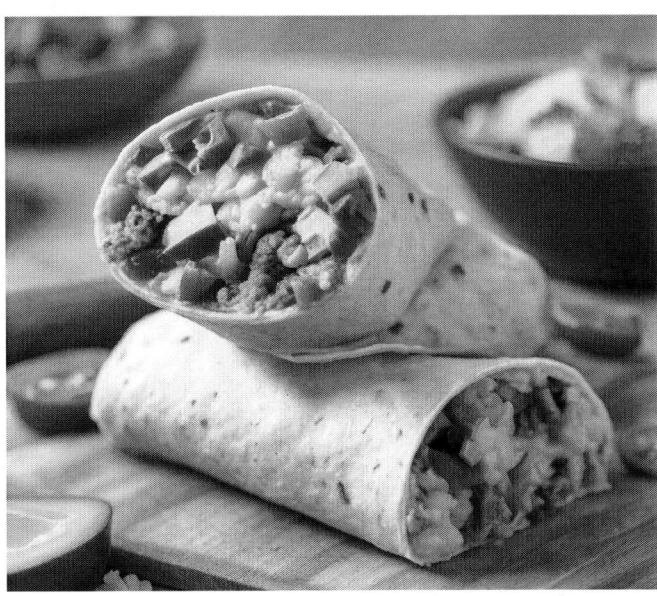

8. Baked Sweet Potato with Yogurt

Ingredients:
- 2 medium sweet potatoes
- 1/2 cup Greek yogurt
- 1 tbsp honey
- 1/4 tsp cinnamon
- 1/4 cup chopped walnuts

Instructions:
1. Preheat the oven to 400°F (200°C). Wash the sweet potatoes and pierce them several times with a fork.
2. Place the sweet potatoes on a baking sheet and bake for 45-60 minutes, or until tender.
3. While the sweet potatoes are baking, mix the Greek yogurt, honey, and cinnamon in a small bowl.
4. Once the sweet potatoes are done, let them cool slightly. Cut them open and fluff the insides with a fork.
5. Top each sweet potato with the yogurt mixture and sprinkle with chopped walnuts.
6. Serve warm.

Nutrition Info (per serving):
- Calories: 250
- Protein: 7g
- Carbohydrates: 45g
- Dietary Fiber: 7g
- Sugars: 20g
- Fat: 6g
- Saturated Fat: 1g
- Cholesterol: 5mg
- Sodium: 60mg

Servings: 2
Cooking Time: 1 hour

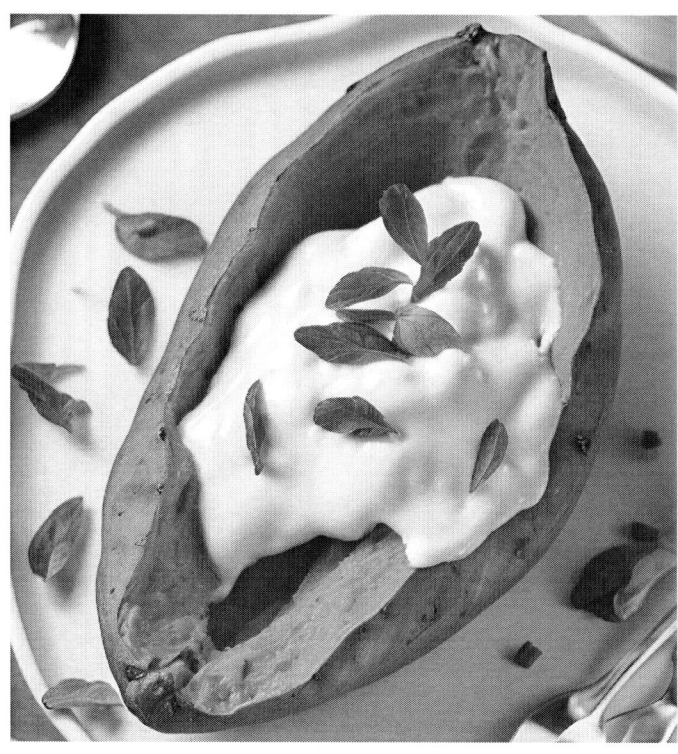

9. Sweet Corn Porridge

Ingredients:
- 1 cup fresh or frozen corn kernels
- 1/2 cup cornmeal
- 2 cups low-fat milk
- 1 cup water
- 1 tbsp honey
- 1/4 tsp nutmeg
- 1 tbsp chopped fresh chives

Instructions:
1. In a saucepan, combine the milk and water and bring to a gentle boil.
2. Slowly whisk in the cornmeal, ensuring there are no lumps.
3. Reduce the heat to low and cook, stirring frequently, for about 15 minutes, or until the mixture thickens.
4. Stir in the corn kernels, honey, and nutmeg, and continue to cook for another 5 minutes.
5. Remove from heat and serve in bowls, garnished with fresh chives.

Nutrition Info (per serving):
- Calories: 220
- Protein: 7g
- Carbohydrates: 38g
- Dietary Fiber: 4g
- Sugars: 10g
- Fat: 4g
- Saturated Fat: 1.5g
- Cholesterol: 10mg
- Sodium: 45mg

Servings: 2
Cooking Time: 25 minutes

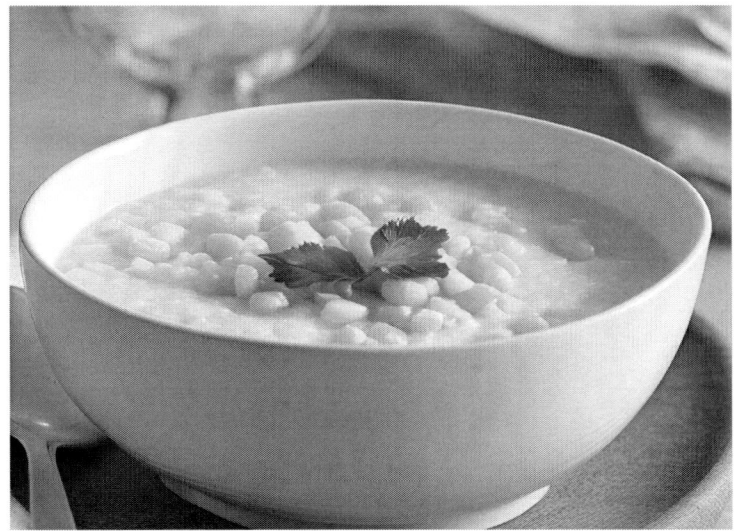

10. Overnight Barley

Ingredients:
- 1 cup pearl barley
- 2 cups low-fat milk
- 1/2 cup water
- 1/4 cup raisins
- 1/4 tsp cinnamon
- 1/4 cup chopped almonds
- 1 tbsp maple syrup
- 1 tsp vanilla extract

Instructions:
1. In a large bowl, combine the pearl barley, milk, water, raisins, cinnamon, and vanilla extract.
2. Cover the bowl and refrigerate overnight.
3. In the morning, transfer the mixture to a saucepan and bring to a simmer over medium heat.
4. Reduce heat to low and cook, stirring occasionally, until the barley is tender and the mixture has thickened, about 20 minutes.
5. Stir in the maple syrup and top with chopped almonds before serving.

Nutrition Info (per serving):
- Calories: 290
- Protein: 9g
- Carbohydrates: 55g
- Dietary Fiber: 8g
- Sugars: 15g
- Fat: 6g
- Saturated Fat: 1g
- Cholesterol: 5mg
- Sodium: 55mg

Servings: 4

Cooking Time: 10 minutes prep + overnight soaking + 20 minutes cooking

11. Gluten-Free Blueberry Waffles

Ingredients:
- 1 cup gluten-free all-purpose flour
- 1 tbsp sugar
- 1 tsp baking powder
- 1/2 tsp baking soda
- 1/2 tsp cinnamon
- 1 cup low-fat milk
- 2 eggs
- 2 tbsp melted coconut oil
- 1 tsp vanilla extract
- 1 cup fresh or frozen blueberries

Instructions:
1. Preheat your waffle iron according to the manufacturer's instructions.
2. In a large bowl, whisk together the gluten-free flour, sugar, baking powder, baking soda, and cinnamon.
3. In another bowl, whisk together the milk, eggs, melted coconut oil, and vanilla extract.
4. Pour the wet ingredients into the dry ingredients and stir until just combined. Gently fold in the blueberries.
5. Lightly grease the waffle iron with cooking spray or a little coconut oil. Pour the batter onto the waffle iron and cook until the waffles are golden brown and crisp, about 3-5 minutes.
6. Serve warm with additional blueberries and a drizzle of honey or maple syrup, if desired.

Nutrition Info (per serving):
- Calories: 220
- Protein: 6g
- Carbohydrates: 34g
- Dietary Fiber: 3g
- Sugars: 10g
- Fat: 7g
- Saturated Fat: 4g
- Cholesterol: 55mg
- Sodium: 210mg

Servings: 4
Cooking Time: 20 minutes

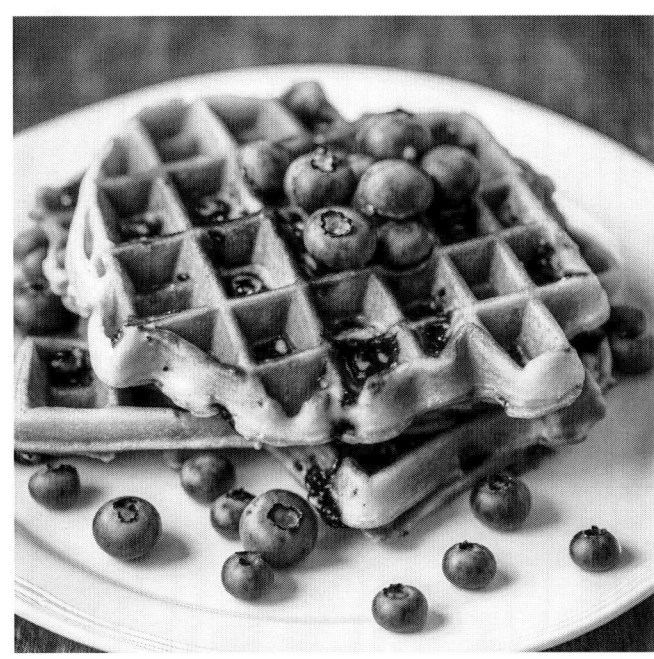

12. Almond Butter Banana Smoothie

Ingredients:
- 1 ripe banana
- 2 tbsp almond butter
- 1 cup unsweetened almond milk
- 1 tbsp honey
- 1/2 tsp cinnamon
- 1/2 tsp vanilla extract
- 1/2 cup ice cubes

Instructions:
1. In a blender, combine the banana, almond butter, almond milk, honey, cinnamon, vanilla extract, and ice cubes.
2. Blend until smooth and creamy.
3. Pour into a glass and serve immediately.

Nutrition Info (per serving):
- Calories: 270
- Protein: 6g
- Carbohydrates: 35g
- Dietary Fiber: 5g
- Sugars: 20g
- Fat: 14g
- Saturated Fat: 1g
- Cholesterol: 0mg
- Sodium: 105mg

Servings: 1
Cooking Time: 5 minutes

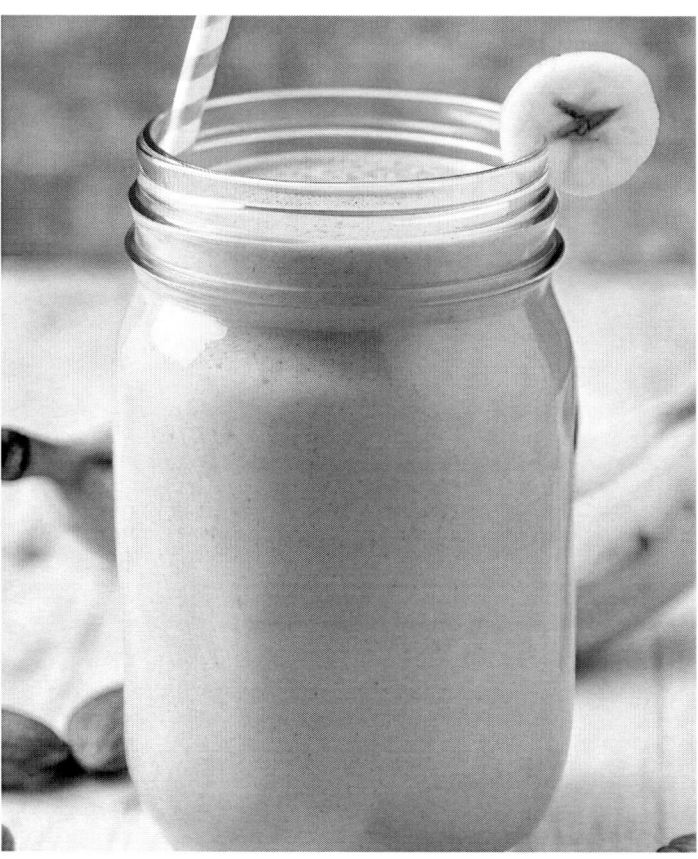

13. Tofu Scramble with Avocado

Ingredients:
- 1 block firm tofu, drained and crumbled
- 1 tbsp olive oil
- 1/2 cup diced bell pepper
- 1/2 cup diced onion
- 1/2 tsp turmeric
- 1/4 tsp black pepper
- 1 avocado, sliced
- 2 tbsp nutritional yeast
- 1/4 cup chopped fresh parsley

Instructions:
1. Heat the olive oil in a large skillet over medium heat. Add the diced bell pepper and onion and cook until softened, about 5 minutes.
2. Add the crumbled tofu, turmeric, and black pepper to the skillet. Cook, stirring frequently, until the tofu is heated through and slightly browned, about 7-10 minutes.
3. Stir in the nutritional yeast and cook for another 2 minutes.
4. Serve the tofu scramble topped with sliced avocado and fresh parsley.

Nutrition Info (per serving):
- Calories: 280
- Protein: 16g
- Carbohydrates: 14g
- Dietary Fiber: 7g
- Sugars: 3g
- Fat: 20g
- Saturated Fat: 3g
- Cholesterol: 0mg
- Sodium: 15mg

Servings: 2
Cooking Time: 15 minutes

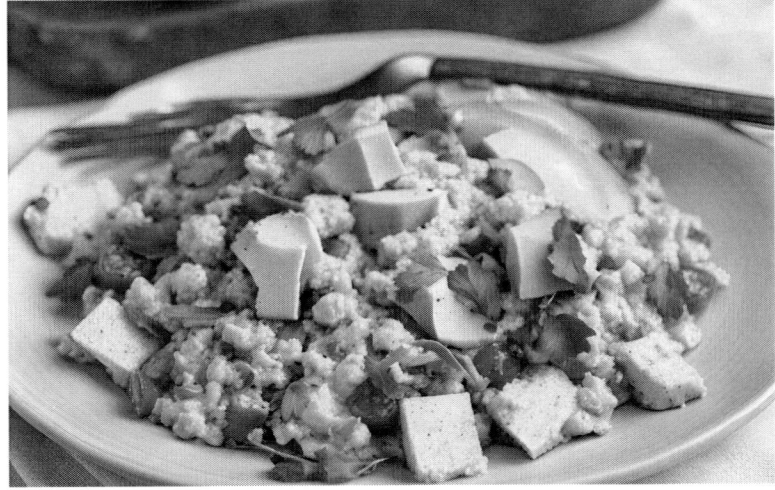

14. Cream of Wheat with Fruit

Ingredients:
- 1/2 cup Cream of Wheat
- 2 cups low-fat milk
- 1 tbsp honey
- 1/2 tsp vanilla extract
- 1/2 cup mixed berries (blueberries, strawberries, raspberries)
- 1 small banana, sliced
- 1/4 tsp cinnamon

Instructions:
1. In a medium saucepan, bring the milk to a gentle boil over medium heat.
2. Gradually whisk in the Cream of Wheat and reduce the heat to low. Cook, stirring constantly, until the mixture thickens, about 3-5 minutes.
3. Remove from heat and stir in the honey and vanilla extract.
4. Serve the Cream of Wheat in bowls topped with mixed berries, banana slices, and a sprinkle of cinnamon.

Nutrition Info (per serving):
- Calories: 230
- Protein: 9g
- Carbohydrates: 40g
- Dietary Fiber: 4g
- Sugars: 20g
- Fat: 5g
- Saturated Fat: 2.5g
- Cholesterol: 10mg
- Sodium: 85mg

Servings: 2
Cooking Time: 10 minutes

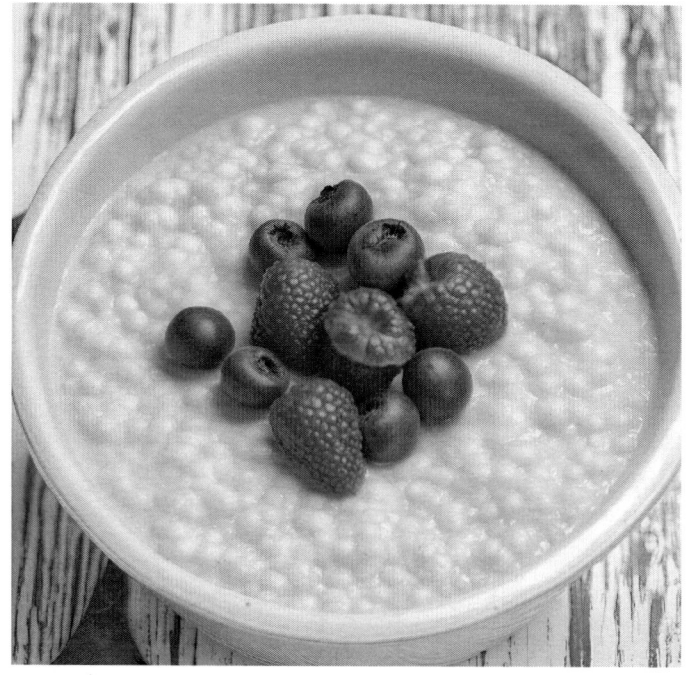

15. Mashed Potato Pancakes

Ingredients:
- 2 cups mashed potatoes (prepared without butter or cream)
- 1/2 cup grated cheddar cheese
- 1/4 cup chopped green onions
- 1 egg, lightly beaten
- 1/4 cup whole wheat flour
- 1 tbsp olive oil for cooking

Instructions:
1. In a large bowl, combine the mashed potatoes, grated cheddar cheese, chopped green onions, beaten egg, and whole wheat flour. Mix until well combined.
2. Heat the olive oil in a large non-stick skillet over medium heat.
3. Scoop about 1/4 cup of the potato mixture and shape it into a patty. Place the patty in the skillet and flatten it slightly with a spatula. Repeat with the remaining mixture.
4. Cook the patties until golden brown and crisp on both sides, about 3-4 minutes per side.
5. Transfer the pancakes to a paper towel-lined plate to drain any excess oil. Serve warm.

Nutrition Info (per serving):
- Calories: 220
- Protein: 8g
- Carbohydrates: 28g
- Dietary Fiber: 3g
- Sugars: 2g
- Fat: 9g
- Saturated Fat: 3g
- Cholesterol: 55mg
- Sodium: 180mg

Servings: 4
Cooking Time: 20 minutes

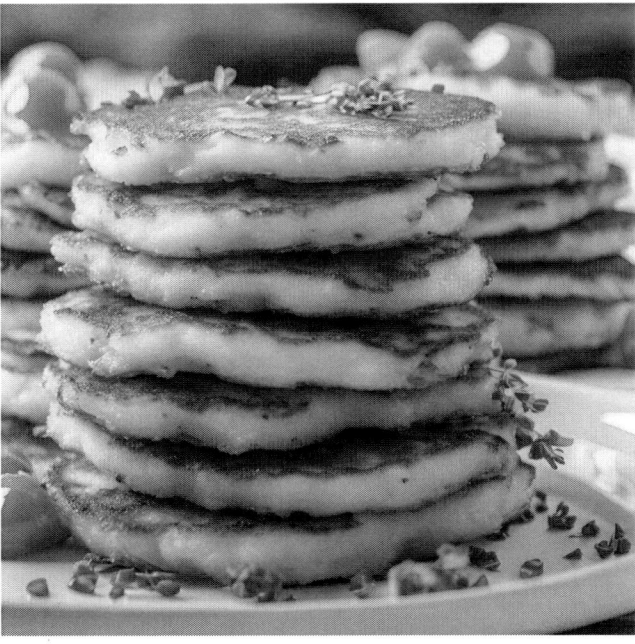

16. Zucchini Bread

Ingredients:
- 2 cups grated zucchini
- 2 cups whole wheat flour
- 1 tsp baking powder
- 1/2 tsp baking soda
- 1 tsp cinnamon
- 1/2 tsp nutmeg
- 2 eggs
- 1/2 cup olive oil
- 1/2 cup honey
- 1 tsp vanilla extract
- 1/2 cup chopped walnuts (optional)

Instructions:
1. Preheat your oven to 350°F (175°C). Grease a 9x5 inch loaf pan.
2. In a large bowl, whisk together the flour, baking powder, baking soda, cinnamon, and nutmeg.
3. In another bowl, beat the eggs, olive oil, honey, and vanilla extract until well combined.
4. Add the grated zucchini to the wet ingredients and mix.
5. Gradually add the dry ingredients to the wet mixture, stirring until just combined. Fold in the walnuts, if using.
6. Pour the batter into the prepared loaf pan and bake for 50-60 minutes, or until a toothpick inserted into the center comes out clean.
7. Let the bread cool in the pan for 10 minutes, then transfer to a wire rack to cool completely before slicing.

Nutrition Info (per serving):
- Calories: 220
- Protein: 4g
- Carbohydrates: 30g
- Dietary Fiber: 3g
- Sugars: 15g
- Fat: 10g
- Saturated Fat: 1.5g
- Cholesterol: 35mg
- Sodium: 95mg

Servings: 10
Cooking Time: 1 hour

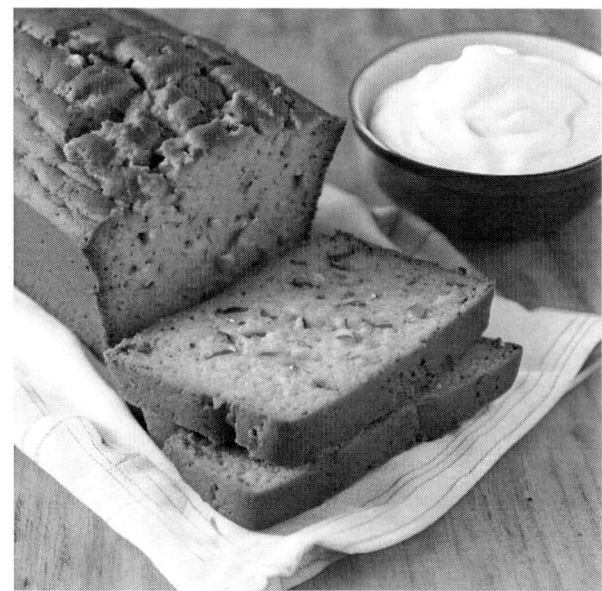

17. Turkey and Spinach Mini Quiches

Ingredients:
- 1/2 lb ground turkey
- 1 cup fresh spinach, chopped
- 1/2 cup diced onion
- 1/2 cup shredded cheddar cheese
- 6 eggs
- 1/4 cup low-fat milk
- 1 tsp garlic powder
- 1/4 tsp black pepper
- 1 tbsp olive oil

Instructions:
1. Preheat your oven to 375°F (190°C). Grease a 12-cup muffin tin.
2. In a skillet, heat the olive oil over medium heat. Add the diced onion and cook until softened, about 5 minutes.
3. Add the ground turkey and cook until no longer pink, breaking it up with a spoon as it cooks.
4. Stir in the chopped spinach and cook until wilted, about 2 minutes.
5. In a large bowl, whisk together the eggs, milk, garlic powder, and black pepper.
6. Divide the turkey and spinach mixture evenly among the muffin cups. Pour the egg mixture over the turkey and spinach, filling each cup about three-quarters full.
7. Sprinkle the shredded cheddar cheese on top.
8. Bake for 20-25 minutes, or until the quiches are set and golden brown.
9. Let the quiches cool in the tin for 5 minutes before removing.

Nutrition Info (per serving):
- Calories: 120
- Protein: 10g
- Carbohydrates: 2g
- Dietary Fiber: 1g
- Sugars: 1g
- Fat: 8g
- Saturated Fat: 3g
- Cholesterol: 135mg
- Sodium: 120mg

Servings: 12
Cooking Time: 30 minutes

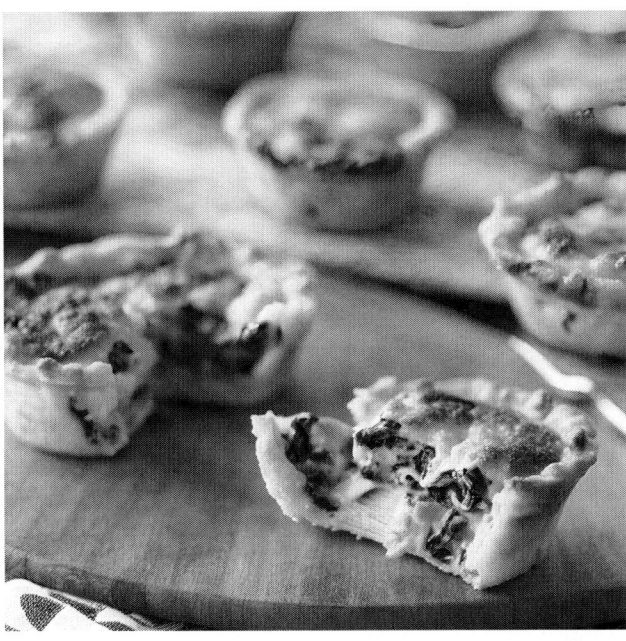

18. Pumpkin Pancakes

Ingredients:
- 1 cup whole wheat flour
- 1 tbsp sugar
- 1 tsp baking powder
- 1/2 tsp baking soda
- 1 tsp cinnamon
- 1/2 tsp nutmeg
- 1/2 tsp ginger
- 1/2 cup pumpkin puree
- 1 cup low-fat milk
- 1 egg
- 2 tbsp melted coconut oil
- 1 tsp vanilla extract

Instructions:
1. In a large bowl, whisk together the flour, sugar, baking powder, baking soda, cinnamon, nutmeg, and ginger.
2. In another bowl, mix the pumpkin puree, milk, egg, melted coconut oil, and vanilla extract until well combined.
3. Pour the wet ingredients into the dry ingredients and stir until just combined.
4. Heat a non-stick skillet or griddle over medium heat. Lightly grease with coconut oil.
5. Pour 1/4 cup of batter onto the skillet for each pancake. Cook until bubbles form on the surface and the edges look set, about 2-3 minutes. Flip and cook for another 2-3 minutes until golden brown.
6. Serve warm with a drizzle of honey or maple syrup.

Nutrition Info (per serving):
- Calories: 150
- Protein: 4g
- Carbohydrates: 23g
- Dietary Fiber: 3g
- Sugars: 5g
- Fat: 5g
- Saturated Fat: 3g
- Cholesterol: 30mg
- Sodium: 170mg

Servings: 8 pancakes
Cooking Time: 20 minutes

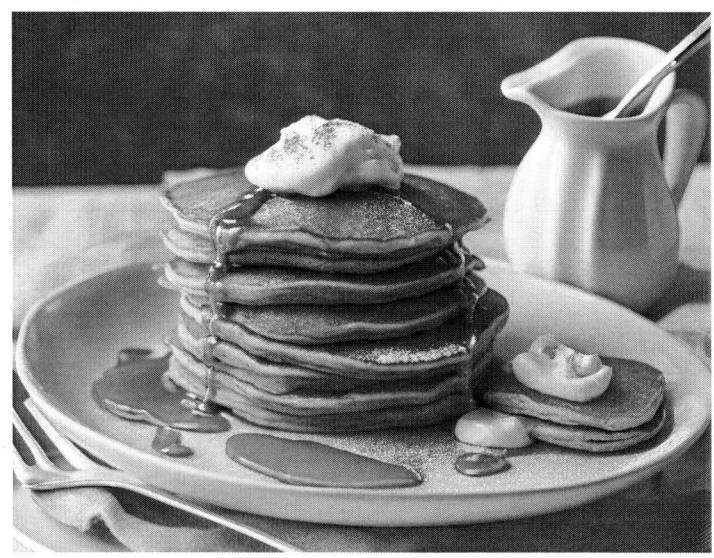

19. Berry Yogurt Parfait

Ingredients:
- 2 cups Greek yogurt
- 1 cup mixed berries (blueberries, strawberries, raspberries)
- 1/4 cup granola
- 2 tbsp honey
- 1/2 tsp vanilla extract

Instructions:
1. In a small bowl, mix the Greek yogurt with the vanilla extract.
2. In serving glasses or bowls, layer 1/4 cup of yogurt, followed by a layer of mixed berries and a sprinkle of granola.
3. Repeat the layers until all ingredients are used, finishing with a drizzle of honey on top.
4. Serve immediately.

Nutrition Info (per serving):
- Calories: 180
- Protein: 10g
- Carbohydrates: 28g
- Dietary Fiber: 4g
- Sugars: 20g
- Fat: 4g
- Saturated Fat: 1.5g
- Cholesterol: 10mg
- Sodium: 55mg

Servings: 2
Cooking Time: 10 minutes

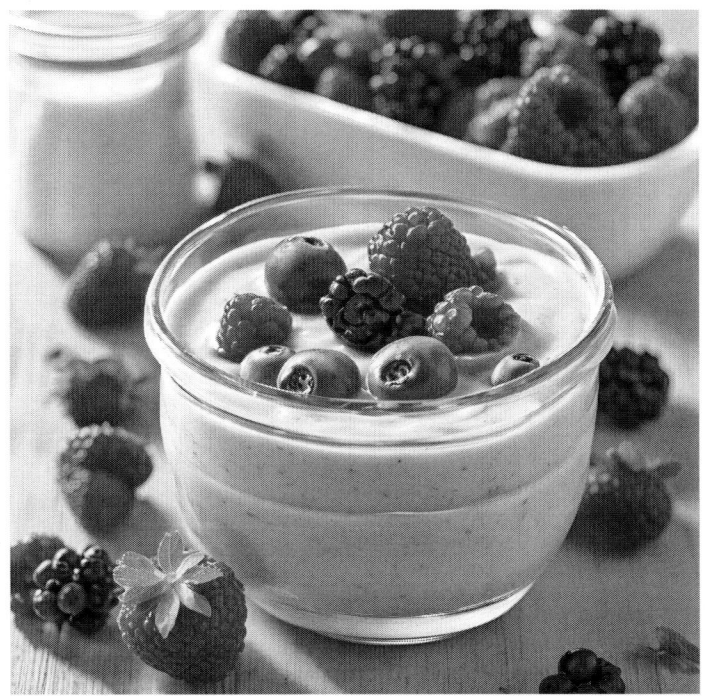

20. Banana Almond Muffins

Ingredients:
- 2 ripe bananas, mashed
- 1/2 cup almond butter
- 2 eggs
- 1/4 cup honey
- 1 tsp vanilla extract
- 1 cup almond flour
- 1/2 tsp baking soda
- 1/2 tsp cinnamon
- 1/4 cup sliced almonds (optional)

Instructions:
1. Preheat your oven to 350°F (175°C). Line a 12-cup muffin tin with paper liners.
2. In a large bowl, mix the mashed bananas, almond butter, eggs, honey, and vanilla extract until well combined.
3. In another bowl, whisk together the almond flour, baking soda, and cinnamon.
4. Add the dry ingredients to the wet ingredients and stir until just combined.
5. Divide the batter evenly among the muffin cups. Sprinkle the tops with sliced almonds, if using.
6. Bake for 20-25 minutes, or until a toothpick inserted into the center of a muffin comes out clean.
7. Let the muffins cool in the tin for 5 minutes, then transfer to a wire rack to cool completely.

Nutrition Info (per serving):
- Calories: 180
- Protein: 6g
- Carbohydrates: 18g
- Dietary Fiber: 3g
- Sugars: 12g
- Fat: 10g
- Saturated Fat: 1g
- Cholesterol: 35mg
- Sodium: 80mg

Servings: 12 muffins
Cooking Time: 30 minutes

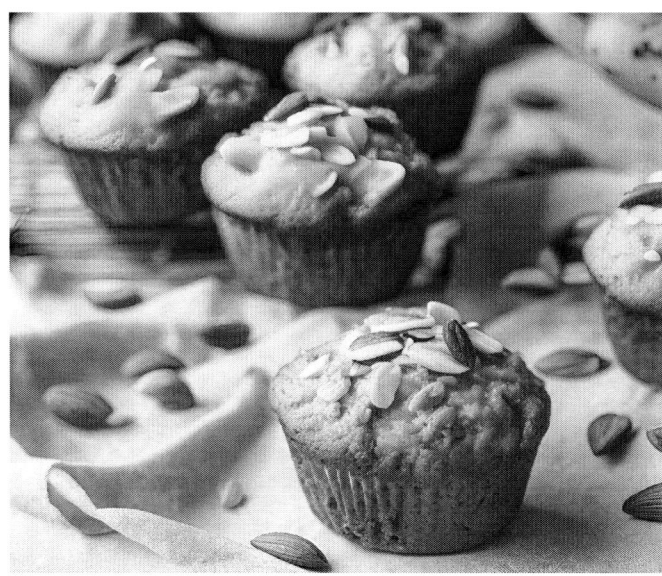

Fish & Seafood Recipes

1. Ginger Salmon Stir-Fry
Ingredients:
- 4 salmon fillets (about 6 oz each)
- 1 tbsp olive oil
- 2 cloves garlic, minced
- 1 tbsp fresh ginger, minced
- 1 red bell pepper, sliced
- 1 yellow bell pepper, sliced
- 1 cup snow peas
- 1 cup broccoli florets
- 1/4 cup low-sodium soy sauce
- 1 tbsp honey
- 1 tsp sesame oil
- 1 tbsp sesame seeds (optional)
- 2 cups cooked brown rice

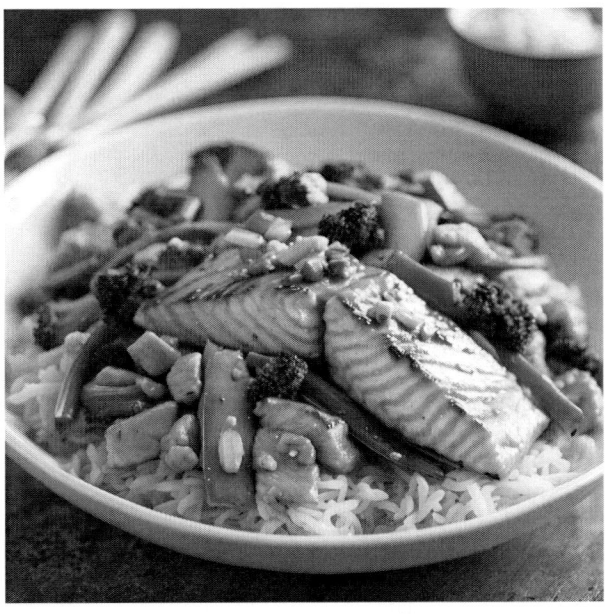

Instructions:
1. Heat the olive oil in a large skillet or wok over medium-high heat. Add the minced garlic and ginger and sauté for 1-2 minutes until fragrant.
2. Add the salmon fillets to the skillet and cook for 3-4 minutes on each side until the salmon is cooked through and flakes easily with a fork. Remove the salmon from the skillet and set aside.
3. In the same skillet, add the sliced bell peppers, snow peas, and broccoli florets. Stir-fry for 5-7 minutes until the vegetables are tender-crisp.
4. In a small bowl, mix the soy sauce, honey, and sesame oil. Pour the sauce over the vegetables and stir to coat evenly.
5. Return the salmon to the skillet, breaking it into large chunks, and gently mix with the vegetables.
6. Sprinkle with sesame seeds, if desired, and serve over cooked brown rice.

Nutrition Info (per serving):
- Calories: 450 Protein: 35g Carbohydrates: 40g Dietary Fiber: 6g
- Sugars: 8g
- Fat: 15g
- Saturated Fat: 2.5g
- Cholesterol: 75mg
- Sodium: 300mg

Servings: 4
Cooking Time: 30 minutes

2. Baked Cod with Lemon and Dill

Ingredients:
- 4 cod fillets (about 6 oz each)
- 2 tbsp olive oil
- 2 tbsp fresh lemon juice
- 2 cloves garlic, minced
- 1 tbsp fresh dill, chopped
- 1 lemon, sliced
- 1/4 tsp paprika

Instructions:
1. Preheat your oven to 400°F (200°C). Line a baking sheet with parchment paper.
2. In a small bowl, mix the olive oil, lemon juice, minced garlic, and chopped dill.
3. Place the cod fillets on the prepared baking sheet. Brush the fillets with the olive oil mixture and sprinkle with paprika.
4. Arrange the lemon slices on top of the fillets.
5. Bake in the preheated oven for 15-20 minutes, or until the fish is opaque and flakes easily with a fork.
6. Serve immediately, garnished with additional fresh dill if desired.

Nutrition Info (per serving):
- Calories: 220
- Protein: 32g
- Carbohydrates: 2g
- Dietary Fiber: 0g
- Sugars: 0g
- Fat: 9g
- Saturated Fat: 1.5g
- Cholesterol: 75mg
- Sodium: 100mg

Servings: 4
Cooking Time: 25 minutes

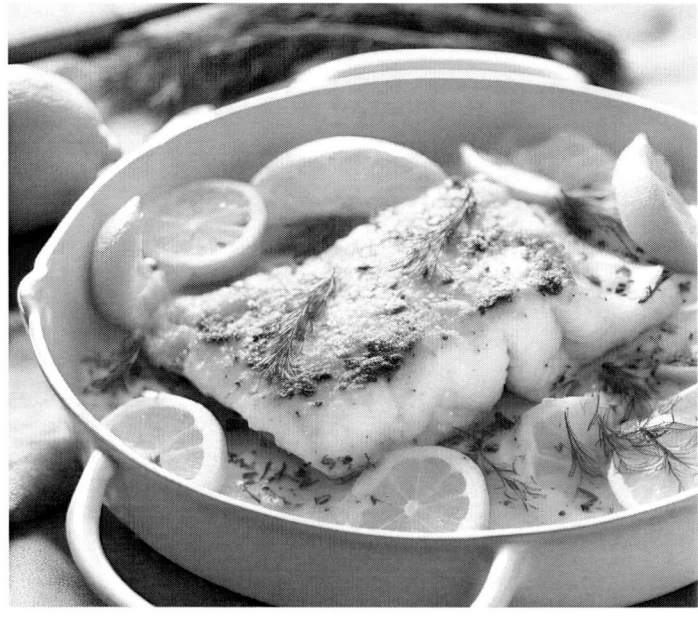

3. Shrimp and Avocado Salad
Ingredients:
- 1 lb cooked shrimp, peeled and deveined
- 2 ripe avocados, diced
- 1 cup cherry tomatoes, halved
- 1/2 red onion, finely chopped
- 1/4 cup fresh cilantro, chopped
- 2 tbsp olive oil
- 2 tbsp fresh lime juice
- 1 tsp cumin
- 1/4 tsp paprika

Instructions:
1. In a large bowl, combine the cooked shrimp, diced avocados, cherry tomatoes, red onion, and fresh cilantro.
2. In a small bowl, whisk together the olive oil, lime juice, cumin, and paprika.
3. Pour the dressing over the shrimp and avocado mixture and toss gently to combine.
4. Serve immediately or chill in the refrigerator for 30 minutes to allow the flavors to meld.

Nutrition Info (per serving):
- Calories: 320
- Protein: 25g
- Carbohydrates: 12g
- Dietary Fiber: 7g
- Sugars: 2g
- Fat: 20g
- Saturated Fat: 3g
- Cholesterol: 190mg
- Sodium: 220mg

Servings: 4
Cooking Time: 15 minutes

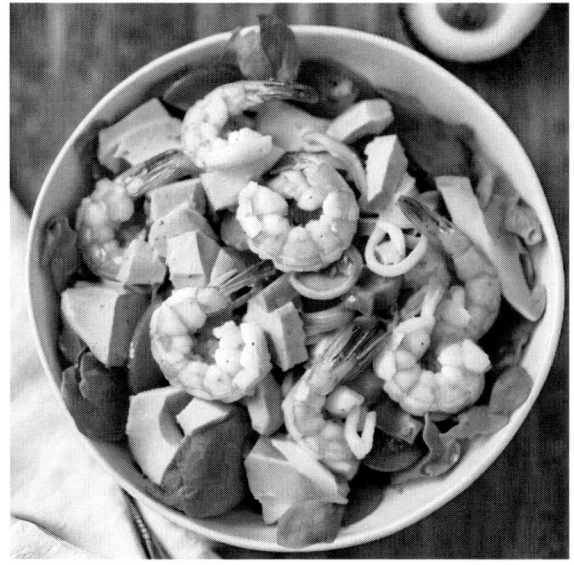

4. Simple Grilled Tilapia

Ingredients:
- 4 tilapia fillets (about 6 oz each)
- 2 tbsp olive oil
- 2 cloves garlic, minced
- 1 tbsp fresh lemon juice
- 1 tsp dried oregano
- 1/4 tsp black pepper
- Lemon wedges, for serving

Instructions:
1. Preheat your grill to medium-high heat.
2. In a small bowl, mix the olive oil, minced garlic, lemon juice, dried oregano, and black pepper.
3. Brush the tilapia fillets with the olive oil mixture on both sides.
4. Place the fillets on the preheated grill and cook for 3-4 minutes on each side, or until the fish is opaque and flakes easily with a fork.
5. Serve immediately with lemon wedges on the side.

Nutrition Info (per serving):
- Calories: 220
- Protein: 30g
- Carbohydrates: 1g
- Dietary Fiber: 0g
- Sugars: 0g
- Fat: 10g
- Saturated Fat: 2g
- Cholesterol: 70mg
- Sodium: 80mg

Servings: 4
Cooking Time: 15 minutes

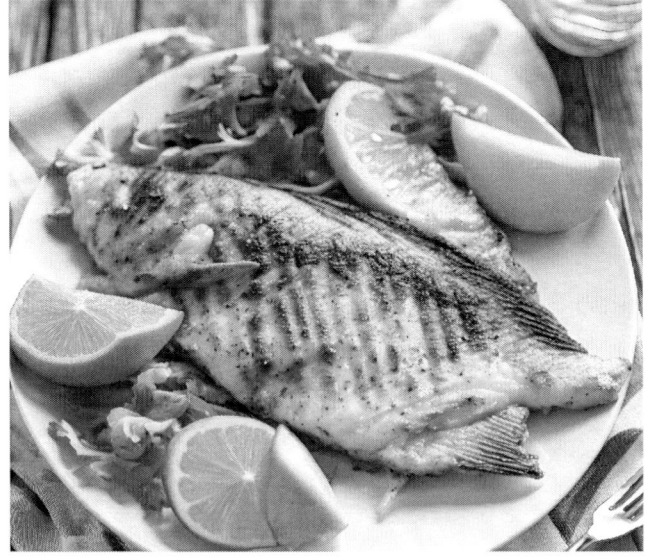

5. Oven-Roasted Trout with Thyme

Ingredients:
- 4 trout fillets (about 6 oz each)
- 2 tbsp olive oil
- 1 lemon, sliced
- 4 sprigs fresh thyme
- 2 cloves garlic, minced
- 1/4 tsp paprika

Instructions:
1. Preheat your oven to 375°F (190°C). Line a baking sheet with parchment paper.
2. Place the trout fillets on the prepared baking sheet. Drizzle with olive oil and sprinkle with minced garlic and paprika.
3. Place a few lemon slices and a sprig of thyme on each fillet.
4. Bake in the preheated oven for 15-20 minutes, or until the fish is opaque and flakes easily with a fork.
5. Serve immediately, garnished with additional fresh thyme if desired.

Nutrition Info (per serving):
- Calories: 250
- Protein: 28g
- Carbohydrates: 2g
- Dietary Fiber: 0g
- Sugars: 0g
- Fat: 14g
- Saturated Fat: 2.5g
- Cholesterol: 70mg
- Sodium: 90mg

Servings: 4
Cooking Time: 25 minutes

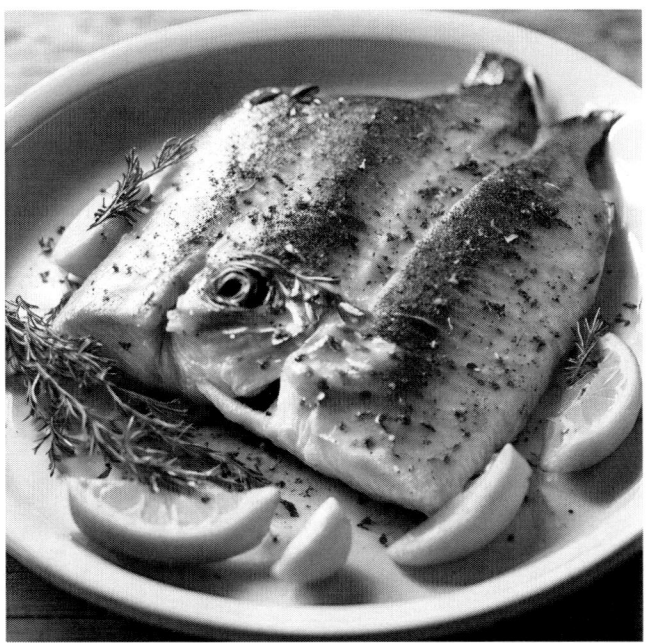

6. Pesto Shrimp Pasta

Ingredients:
- 1 lb large shrimp, peeled and deveined
- 8 oz whole wheat pasta
- 1 cup cherry tomatoes, halved
- 1/2 cup prepared pesto sauce
- 1 tbsp olive oil
- 2 cloves garlic, minced
- 1/4 cup grated Parmesan cheese
- 1/4 tsp red pepper flakes (optional)
- Fresh basil leaves for garnish

Instructions:
1. Cook the pasta according to the package instructions. Drain and set aside.
2. In a large skillet, heat the olive oil over medium heat. Add the minced garlic and cook for 1-2 minutes until fragrant.
3. Add the shrimp to the skillet and cook until pink and opaque, about 3-4 minutes.
4. Add the cherry tomatoes and cook for another 2 minutes until softened.
5. Stir in the cooked pasta and pesto sauce, mixing until well combined and heated through.
6. Sprinkle with grated Parmesan cheese and red pepper flakes, if using.
7. Serve immediately, garnished with fresh basil leaves.

Nutrition Info (per serving):
- Calories: 400
- Protein: 30g
- Carbohydrates: 40g
- Dietary Fiber: 6g
- Sugars: 4g
- Fat: 14g
- Saturated Fat: 3g
- Cholesterol: 180mg
- Sodium: 450mg

Servings: 4
Cooking Time: 25 minutes

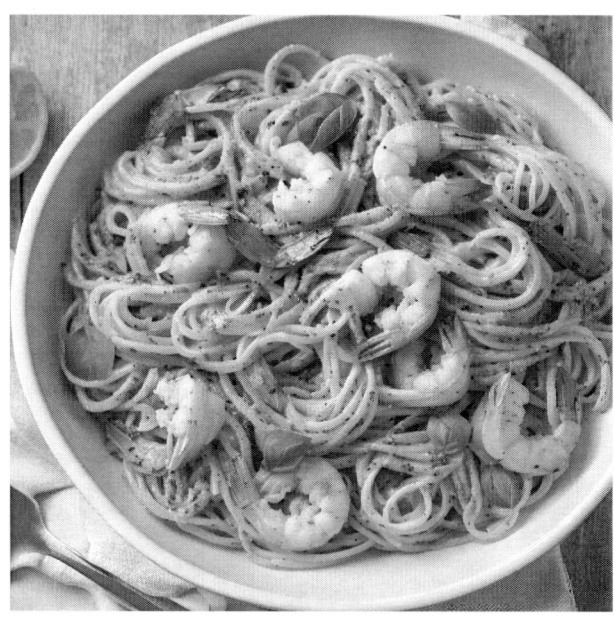

7. Clam Soup with Vegetables

Ingredients:
- 2 dozen clams, cleaned
- 1 tbsp olive oil
- 1 onion, diced
- 2 carrots, diced
- 2 celery stalks, diced
- 2 cloves garlic, minced
- 4 cups low-sodium vegetable broth
- 1 cup diced potatoes
- 1/2 cup chopped fresh parsley
- 1/2 tsp thyme
- 1/4 tsp paprika

Instructions:
1. In a large pot, heat the olive oil over medium heat. Add the diced onion, carrots, and celery, and cook until softened, about 5-7 minutes.
2. Add the minced garlic and cook for another 1-2 minutes.
3. Pour in the vegetable broth and bring to a boil. Add the diced potatoes, thyme, and paprika, and simmer until the potatoes are tender, about 10 minutes.
4. Add the clams to the pot and cover. Cook for 5-7 minutes, or until the clams open. Discard any clams that do not open.
5. Stir in the chopped parsley and serve immediately.

Nutrition Info (per serving):
- Calories: 250
- Protein: 20g
- Carbohydrates: 28g
- Dietary Fiber: 5g
- Sugars: 6g
- Fat: 7g
- Saturated Fat: 1g
- Cholesterol: 50mg
- Sodium: 320mg

Servings: 4
Cooking Time: 35 minutes

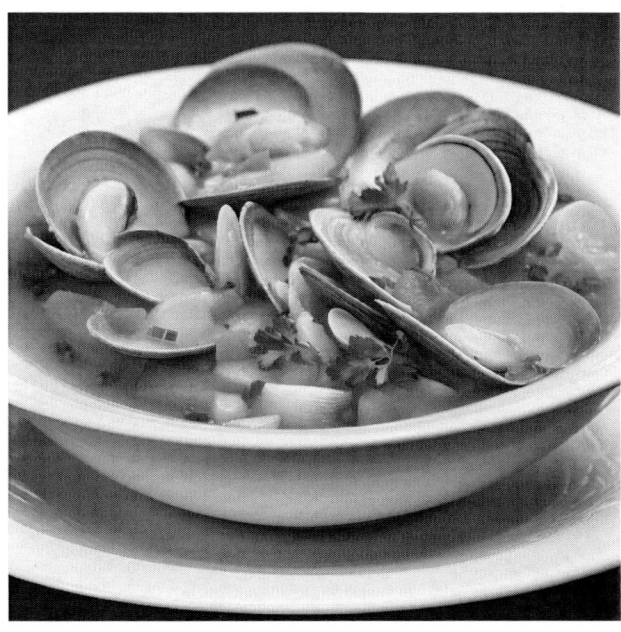

8. Crab and Spinach Stuffed Mushrooms

Ingredients:
- 16 large mushroom caps, stems removed and cleaned
- 1 cup cooked crab meat
- 1 cup fresh spinach, chopped
- 1/2 cup ricotta cheese
- 1/4 cup grated Parmesan cheese
- 1 clove garlic, minced
- 1 tbsp olive oil
- 1/4 tsp paprika

Instructions:
1. Preheat your oven to 375°F (190°C). Line a baking sheet with parchment paper.
2. In a skillet, heat the olive oil over medium heat. Add the minced garlic and chopped spinach, and cook until the spinach is wilted, about 2-3 minutes.
3. In a bowl, mix together the cooked spinach, crab meat, ricotta cheese, Parmesan cheese, and paprika.
4. Spoon the mixture into the mushroom caps, distributing evenly.
5. Place the stuffed mushrooms on the prepared baking sheet and bake for 20 minutes, or until the mushrooms are tender and the filling is heated through.
6. Serve warm.

Nutrition Info (per serving):
- Calories: 120
- Protein: 10g
- Carbohydrates: 6g
- Dietary Fiber: 1g
- Sugars: 2g
- Fat: 7g
- Saturated Fat: 2g
- Cholesterol: 30mg
- Sodium: 180mg

Servings: 4
Cooking Time: 30 minutes

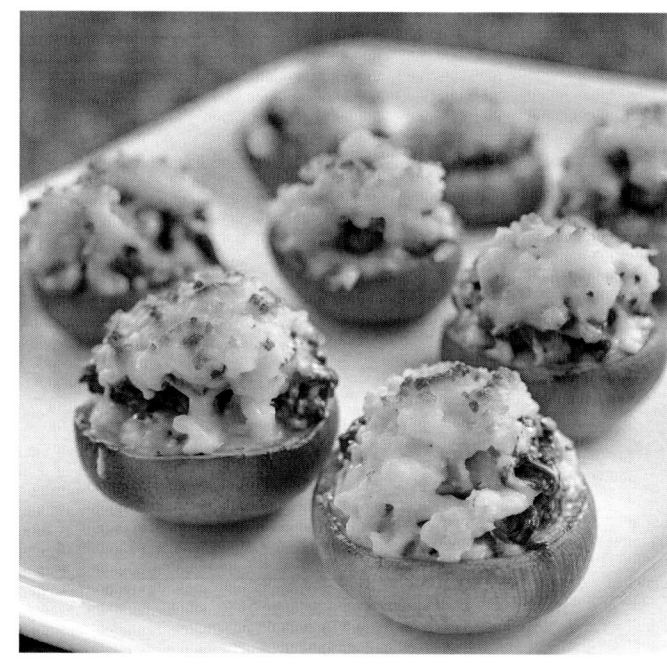

9. Mild White Fish Soup

Ingredients:
- 1 lb mild white fish fillets (such as cod or haddock), cut into chunks
- 1 tbsp olive oil
- 1 onion, diced
- 2 carrots, diced
- 2 celery stalks, diced
- 2 cloves garlic, minced
- 4 cups low-sodium chicken broth
- 1 cup diced potatoes
- 1/2 cup diced tomatoes
- 1/4 cup chopped fresh dill
- 1/2 tsp thyme
- 1/4 tsp paprika

Instructions:
1. In a large pot, heat the olive oil over medium heat. Add the diced onion, carrots, and celery, and cook until softened, about 5-7 minutes.
2. Add the minced garlic and cook for another 1-2 minutes.
3. Pour in the chicken broth and bring to a boil. Add the diced potatoes, tomatoes, thyme, and paprika, and simmer until the potatoes are tender, about 10 minutes.
4. Add the fish chunks to the pot and cook for 5-7 minutes, or until the fish is opaque and cooked through.
5. Stir in the chopped dill and serve immediately.

Nutrition Info (per serving):
- Calories: 240
- Protein: 25g
- Carbohydrates: 22g
- Dietary Fiber: 4g
- Sugars: 5g
- Fat: 7g
- Saturated Fat: 1g
- Cholesterol: 55mg
- Sodium: 270mg

Servings: 4
Cooking Time: 35 minutes

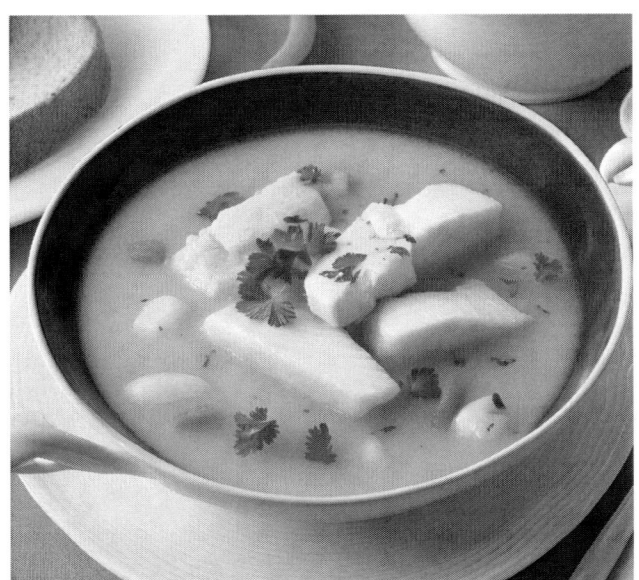

10. Salmon and Rice Casserole

Ingredients:
- 1 lb salmon fillets, cooked and flaked
- 2 cups cooked brown rice
- 1 cup steamed broccoli florets
- 1/2 cup shredded cheddar cheese
- 1/2 cup low-fat milk
- 1/4 cup Greek yogurt
- 1 egg, beaten
- 1 tbsp olive oil
- 2 cloves garlic, minced
- 1/4 tsp paprika

Instructions:
1. Preheat your oven to 350°F (175°C). Grease a 9x9 inch baking dish.
2. In a skillet, heat the olive oil over medium heat. Add the minced garlic and cook for 1-2 minutes until fragrant.
3. In a large bowl, combine the cooked salmon, cooked brown rice, steamed broccoli, shredded cheddar cheese, and the garlic mixture.
4. In a separate bowl, whisk together the milk, Greek yogurt, beaten egg, and paprika.
5. Pour the milk mixture over the salmon and rice mixture and stir until well combined.
6. Transfer the mixture to the prepared baking dish and spread evenly.
7. Bake for 25-30 minutes, or until the casserole is heated through and the top is golden brown.
8. Let cool for 5 minutes before serving.

Nutrition Info (per serving):
- Calories: 350
- Protein: 28g
- Carbohydrates: 30g
- Dietary Fiber: 4g
- Sugars: 4g
- Fat: 14g
- Saturated Fat: 4g
- Cholesterol: 100mg
- Sodium: 180mg

Servings: 4
Cooking Time: 40 minutes

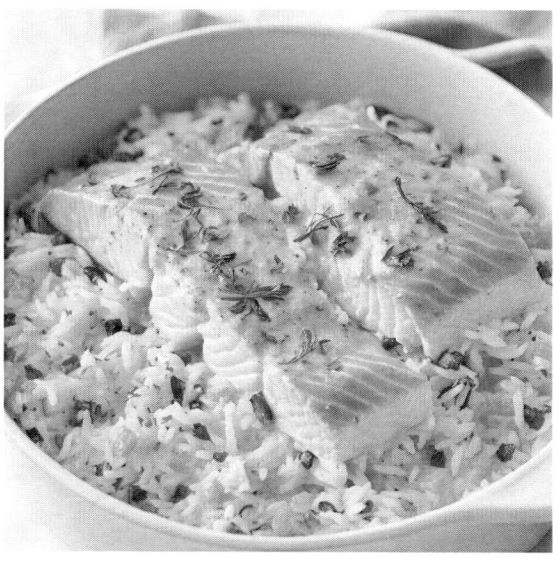

11. Steamed Scallops with Ginger

Ingredients:
- 1 lb sea scallops
- 2 tbsp fresh ginger, julienned
- 2 cloves garlic, minced
- 2 tbsp low-sodium soy sauce
- 1 tbsp rice vinegar
- 1 tbsp sesame oil
- 2 green onions, sliced
- 1/4 tsp red pepper flakes (optional)

Instructions:
1. Rinse the scallops and pat dry with paper towels.
2. Arrange the scallops in a single layer on a heatproof plate or steamer basket.
3. In a small bowl, mix the ginger, garlic, soy sauce, rice vinegar, and sesame oil.
4. Pour the sauce mixture over the scallops.
5. Steam the scallops over simmering water for 5-7 minutes, or until they are opaque and cooked through.
6. Garnish with sliced green onions and red pepper flakes (if using) before serving.

Nutrition Info (per serving):
- Calories: 190
- Protein: 22g
- Carbohydrates: 6g
- Dietary Fiber: 1g
- Sugars: 0g
- Fat: 9g
- Saturated Fat: 1g
- Cholesterol: 35mg
- Sodium: 350mg

Servings: 4
 Cooking Time: 15 minutes

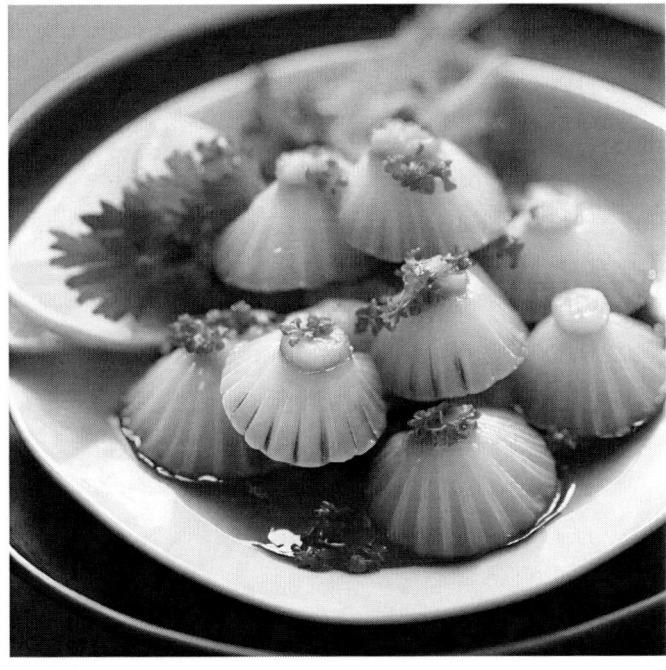

12. Poached Haddock in Milk

Ingredients:
- 1 lb haddock fillets
- 2 cups low-fat milk
- 1 small onion, thinly sliced
- 1 bay leaf
- 1/4 tsp paprika
- 1 tbsp fresh parsley, chopped

Instructions:
1. In a large skillet, combine the milk, onion, bay leaf, and paprika. Bring to a simmer over medium heat.
2. Add the haddock fillets to the skillet, ensuring they are submerged in the milk.
3. Poach the fish for 8-10 minutes, or until it is opaque and flakes easily with a fork.
4. Remove the fillets from the skillet with a slotted spoon and place them on a serving dish.
5. Strain the poaching liquid, discarding the solids.
6. Drizzle a little of the strained poaching liquid over the fish and garnish with chopped parsley before serving.

Nutrition Info (per serving):
- Calories: 220
- Protein: 30g
- Carbohydrates: 10g
- Dietary Fiber: 1g
- Sugars: 8g
- Fat: 7g
- Saturated Fat: 4g
- Cholesterol: 75mg
- Sodium: 140mg

Servings: 4
Cooking Time: 20 minutes

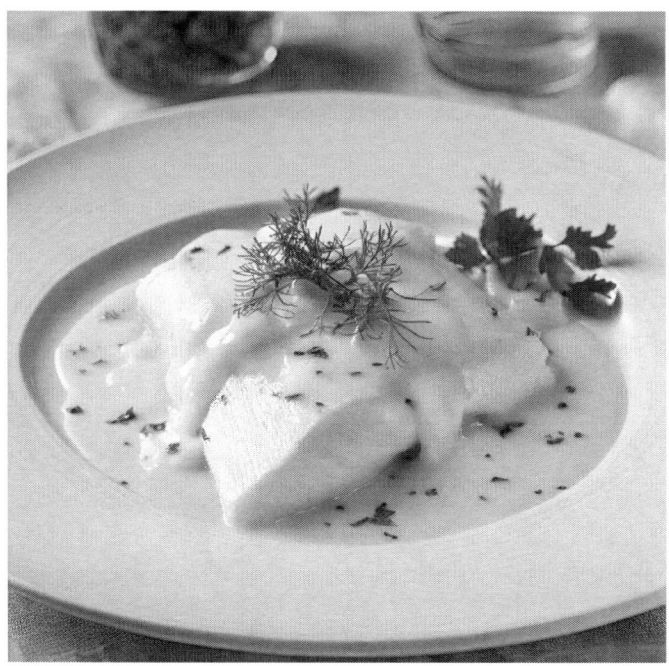

13. Baked Tilapia with Oats Crust

Ingredients:
- 4 tilapia fillets (about 6 oz each)
- 1/2 cup rolled oats
- 1/4 cup grated Parmesan cheese
- 2 tbsp fresh parsley, chopped
- 1/2 tsp paprika
- 1/4 tsp garlic powder
- 1/4 cup Greek yogurt
- 1 tbsp lemon juice
- 1 tbsp olive oil

Instructions:
1. Preheat your oven to 400°F (200°C). Line a baking sheet with parchment paper.
2. In a food processor, pulse the rolled oats until coarsely ground. Transfer to a bowl and mix with Parmesan cheese, chopped parsley, paprika, and garlic powder.
3. In another bowl, mix the Greek yogurt and lemon juice.
4. Brush the tilapia fillets with the yogurt mixture, then coat them with the oat mixture, pressing gently to adhere.
5. Place the coated fillets on the prepared baking sheet and drizzle with olive oil.
6. Bake for 15-20 minutes, or until the fish is opaque and flakes easily with a fork.
7. Serve immediately.

Nutrition Info (per serving):
- Calories: 300
- Protein: 35g
- Carbohydrates: 12g
- Dietary Fiber: 2g
- Sugars: 2g
- Fat: 12g
- Saturated Fat: 3g
- Cholesterol: 80mg
- Sodium: 200mg

Servings: 4
Cooking Time: 25 minutes

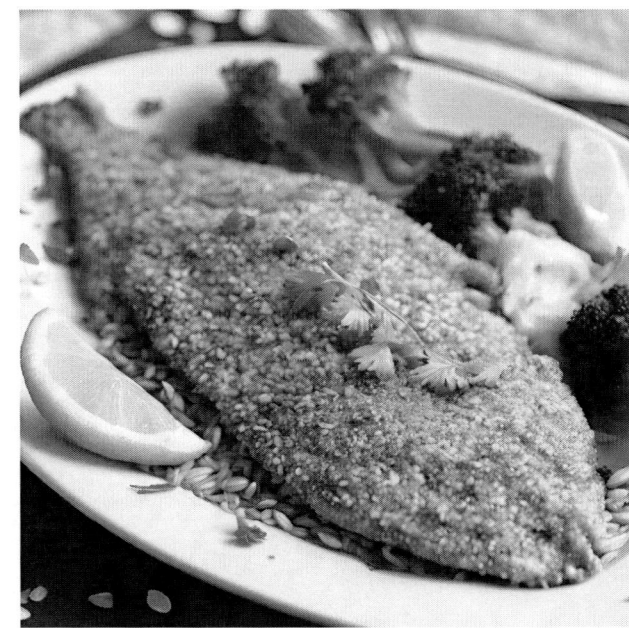

14. Crab Salad with Light Mayo

Ingredients:
- 1 lb lump crab meat
- 1/2 cup light mayonnaise
- 1 tbsp Dijon mustard
- 1 tbsp lemon juice
- 1 celery stalk, finely chopped
- 1/4 cup red bell pepper, finely chopped
- 2 green onions, finely chopped
- 1 tbsp fresh dill, chopped

Instructions:
1. In a large bowl, combine the light mayonnaise, Dijon mustard, and lemon juice.
2. Add the crab meat, celery, red bell pepper, green onions, and chopped dill to the bowl.
3. Gently mix all ingredients until well combined.
4. Chill the salad in the refrigerator for at least 30 minutes before serving.
5. Serve on a bed of lettuce or with whole grain crackers.

Nutrition Info (per serving):
- Calories: 200
- Protein: 25g
- Carbohydrates: 6g
- Dietary Fiber: 1g
- Sugars: 3g
- Fat: 8g
- Saturated Fat: 1g
- Cholesterol: 85mg
- Sodium: 460mg

Servings: 4

Cooking Time: 10 minutes + 30 minutes chilling

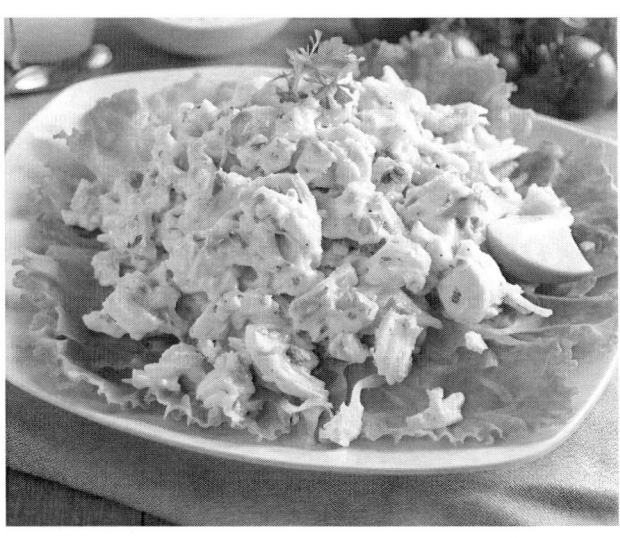

15. Mackerel Pate

Ingredients:
- 8 oz smoked mackerel fillets, skin removed and flaked
- 1/4 cup Greek yogurt
- 2 tbsp light cream cheese
- 1 tbsp lemon juice
- 1 tbsp fresh dill, chopped
- 1 tsp horseradish sauce
- 1/4 tsp paprika

Instructions:
1. In a food processor, combine the flaked mackerel, Greek yogurt, light cream cheese, lemon juice, chopped dill, horseradish sauce, and paprika.
2. Blend until smooth and creamy.
3. Transfer the pate to a bowl and chill in the refrigerator for at least 1 hour before serving.
4. Serve with whole grain crackers or vegetable sticks.

Nutrition Info (per serving):
- Calories: 150
- Protein: 15g
- Carbohydrates: 2g
- Dietary Fiber: 0g
- Sugars: 1g
- Fat: 9g
- Saturated Fat: 2g
- Cholesterol: 30mg
- Sodium: 190mg

Servings: 4
Cooking Time: 10 minutes + 1 hour chilling

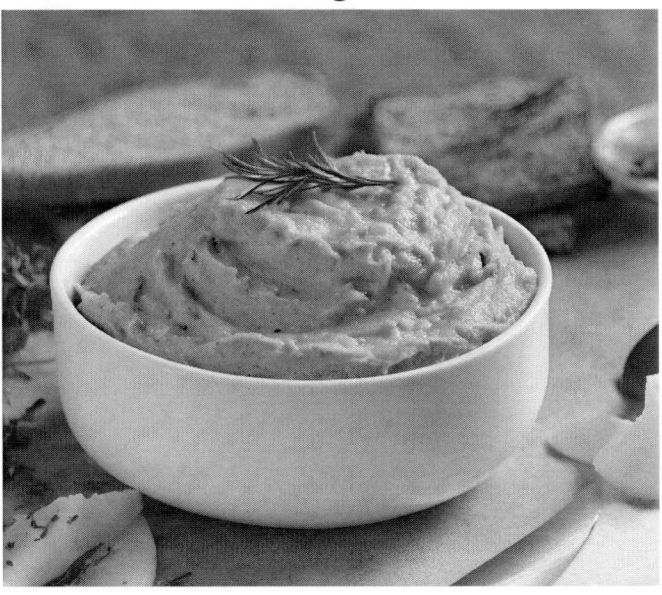

16. Grilled Salmon with Mango Salsa

Ingredients:
- 4 salmon fillets (about 6 oz each)
- 1 tbsp olive oil
- 1/2 tsp paprika
- 1 ripe mango, diced
- 1/2 red bell pepper, diced
- 1/4 cup red onion, finely chopped
- 1/4 cup fresh cilantro, chopped
- 2 tbsp lime juice

Instructions:
1. Preheat your grill to medium-high heat.
2. Brush the salmon fillets with olive oil and sprinkle with paprika.
3. Grill the salmon for 4-5 minutes on each side, or until it flakes easily with a fork.
4. While the salmon is grilling, prepare the mango salsa by combining the diced mango, red bell pepper, red onion, cilantro, and lime juice in a bowl.
5. Serve the grilled salmon topped with the mango salsa.

Nutrition Info (per serving):
- Calories: 350
- Protein: 32g
- Carbohydrates: 15g
- Dietary Fiber: 3g
- Sugars: 12g
- Fat: 18g
- Saturated Fat: 3g
- Cholesterol: 85mg
- Sodium: 70mg

Servings: 4
 Cooking Time: 20 minutes

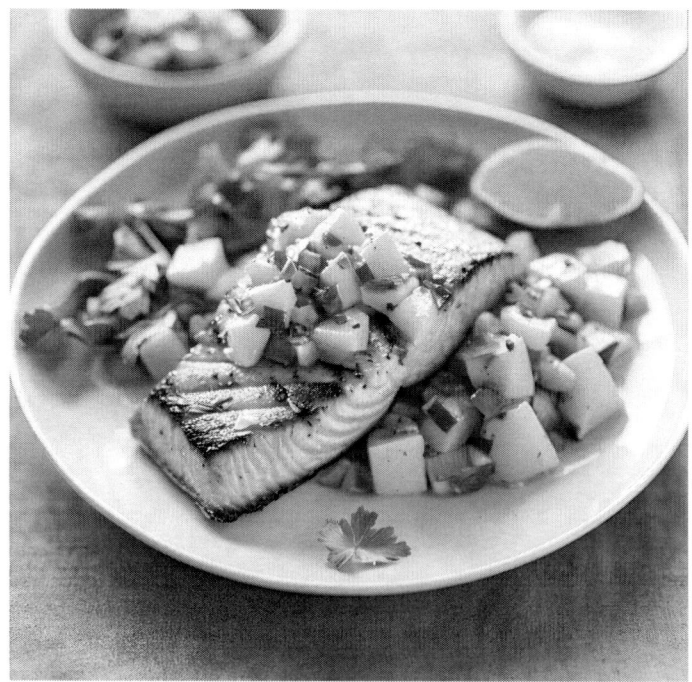

17. Sea Bass with Roasted Vegetables

Ingredients:
- 4 sea bass fillets (about 6 oz each)
- 1 tbsp olive oil
- 1 tsp thyme
- 1 zucchini, sliced
- 1 yellow squash, sliced
- 1 red bell pepper, sliced
- 1 red onion, sliced
- 1 tbsp balsamic vinegar
- 1/4 tsp paprika

Instructions:
1. Preheat your oven to 400°F (200°C). Line a baking sheet with parchment paper.
2. In a large bowl, toss the sliced zucchini, yellow squash, red bell pepper, and red onion with olive oil, balsamic vinegar, thyme, and paprika.
3. Spread the vegetables in a single layer on the prepared baking sheet.
4. Roast the vegetables for 20 minutes.
5. While the vegetables are roasting, heat a non-stick skillet over medium-high heat. Cook the sea bass fillets for 3-4 minutes on each side, or until they are opaque and flake easily with a fork.
6. Serve the sea bass with the roasted vegetables.

Nutrition Info (per serving):
- Calories: 280
- Protein: 32g
- Carbohydrates: 12g
- Dietary Fiber: 3g
- Sugars: 6g
- Fat: 12g
- Saturated Fat: 2g
- Cholesterol: 70mg
- Sodium: 85mg

Servings: 4
Cooking Time: 30 minutes

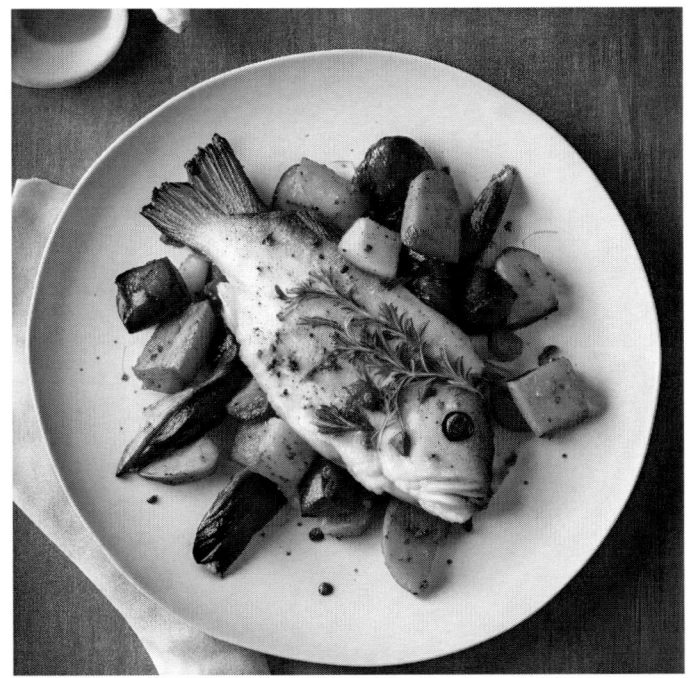

18. Shrimp and Spinach Quiche

Ingredients:
- 1 pre-made whole wheat pie crust
- 1 lb large shrimp, peeled and deveined
- 2 cups fresh spinach, chopped
- 1/2 cup shredded Swiss cheese
- 4 eggs
- 1 cup low-fat milk
- 1 tsp garlic powder
- 1/4 tsp paprika

Instructions:
1. Preheat your oven to 375°F (190°C).
2. Place the pie crust in a 9-inch pie dish and set aside.
3. In a skillet, cook the shrimp over medium heat until pink and opaque, about 3-4 minutes. Remove from heat and chop into bite-sized pieces.
4. In a large bowl, whisk together the eggs, milk, garlic powder, and paprika.
5. Spread the chopped spinach and shrimp evenly in the pie crust. Sprinkle with shredded Swiss cheese.
6. Pour the egg mixture over the spinach and shrimp.
7. Bake for 35-40 minutes, or until the quiche is set and golden brown on top.
8. Let the quiche cool for 5 minutes before slicing and serving.

Nutrition Info (per serving):
- Calories: 290
- Protein: 22g
- Carbohydrates: 16g
- Dietary Fiber: 2g
- Sugars: 3g
- Fat: 15g
- Saturated Fat: 5g
- Cholesterol: 240mg
- Sodium: 330mg

Servings: 6
Cooking Time: 50 minutes

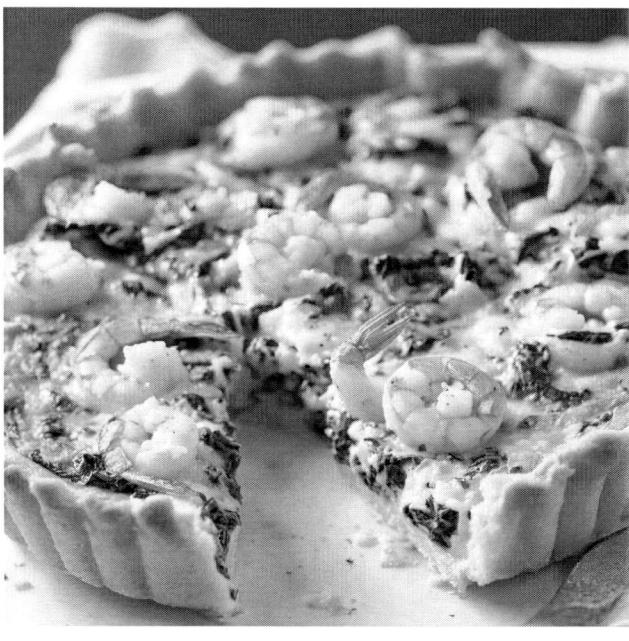

19. Parmesan Crusted Halibut

Ingredients:
- 4 halibut fillets (about 6 oz each)
- 1/2 cup grated Parmesan cheese
- 1/4 cup whole wheat bread crumbs
- 2 tbsp olive oil
- 1 tbsp lemon juice
- 1 tsp garlic powder
- 1/4 tsp paprika

Instructions:
1. Preheat your oven to 400°F (200°C). Line a baking sheet with parchment paper.
2. In a bowl, mix the grated Parmesan cheese, whole wheat bread crumbs, garlic powder, and paprika.
3. Brush the halibut fillets with olive oil and lemon juice.
4. Press the Parmesan mixture onto the top of each fillet.
5. Place the fillets on the prepared baking sheet and bake for 12-15 minutes, or until the fish is opaque and flakes easily with a fork.
6. Serve immediately.

Nutrition Info (per serving):
- Calories: 320
- Protein: 35g
- Carbohydrates: 6g
- Dietary Fiber: 1g
- Sugars: 0g
- Fat: 18g
- Saturated Fat: 5g
- Cholesterol: 75mg
- Sodium: 250mg

Servings: 4
Cooking Time: 20 minutes

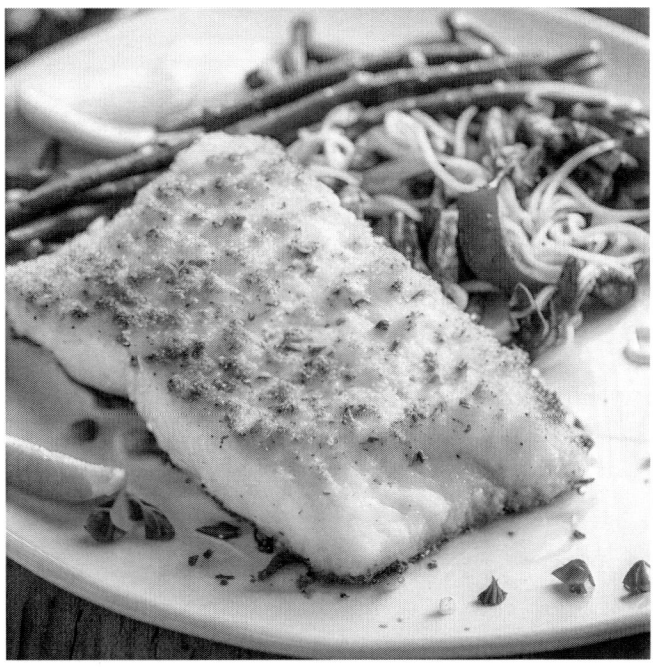

20. Tuna Steak with Tomato Salsa

Ingredients:
- 4 tuna steaks (about 6 oz each)
- 1 tbsp olive oil
- 1 tsp dried oregano
- 1 cup cherry tomatoes, halved
- 1/4 cup red onion, finely chopped
- 1/4 cup fresh cilantro, chopped
- 2 tbsp lime juice
- 1/4 tsp cumin

Instructions:
1. Preheat your grill to medium-high heat.
2. Brush the tuna steaks with olive oil and sprinkle with dried oregano.
3. Grill the tuna steaks for 3-4 minutes on each side, or until they are seared on the outside and slightly pink in the center.
4. While the tuna is grilling, prepare the tomato salsa by combining the cherry tomatoes, red onion, cilantro, lime juice, and cumin in a bowl.
5. Serve the grilled tuna steaks topped with the tomato salsa.

Nutrition Info (per serving):
- Calories: 300
- Protein: 38g
- Carbohydrates: 6g
- Dietary Fiber: 2g
- Sugars: 3g
- Fat: 14g
- Saturated Fat: 2.5g
- Cholesterol: 70mg
- Sodium: 85mg

Servings: 4
 Cooking Time: 20 minutes

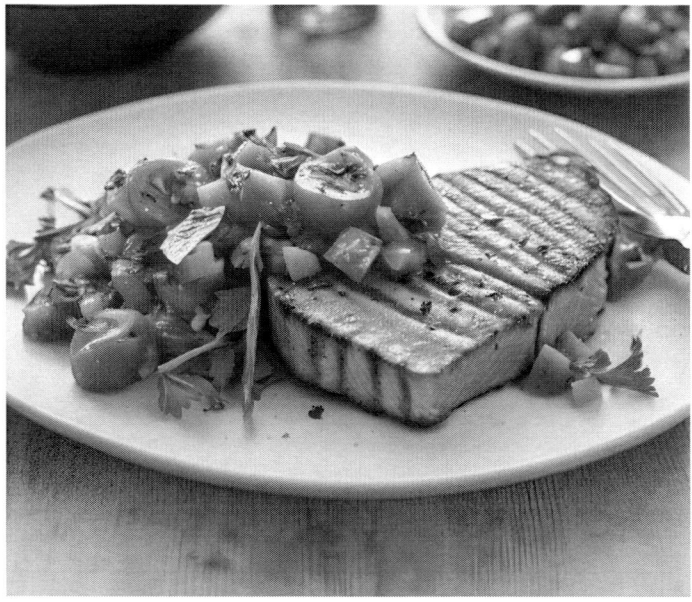

21. Fish Fillet with Light Dill Sauce

Ingredients:
- 4 white fish fillets (such as cod or haddock, about 6 oz each)
- 1 tbsp olive oil
- 1/2 cup low-fat Greek yogurt
- 2 tbsp fresh dill, chopped
- 1 tbsp lemon juice
- 1 clove garlic, minced
- 1/4 tsp paprika

Instructions:
1. Preheat your oven to 375°F (190°C). Line a baking sheet with parchment paper.
2. Brush the fish fillets with olive oil and place them on the prepared baking sheet.
3. Bake the fish for 15-20 minutes, or until it is opaque and flakes easily with a fork.
4. While the fish is baking, prepare the dill sauce by combining the Greek yogurt, fresh dill, lemon juice, minced garlic, and paprika in a bowl.
5. Serve the baked fish fillets topped with the light dill sauce.

Nutrition Info (per serving):
- Calories: 220
- Protein: 32g
- Carbohydrates: 4g
- Dietary Fiber: 0g
- Sugars: 2g
- Fat: 8g
- Saturated Fat: 2g
- Cholesterol: 70mg
- Sodium: 85mg

Servings: 4
Cooking Time: 25 minutes

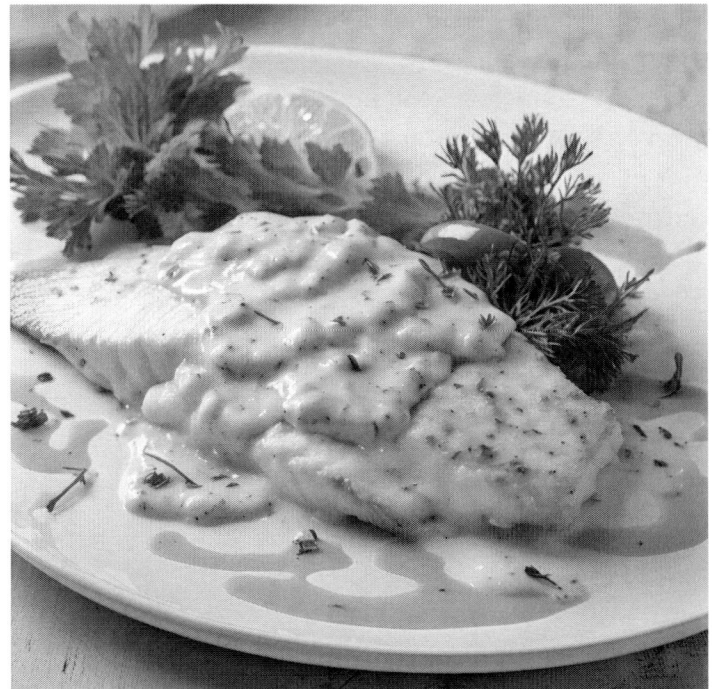

Poultry Recipes

1. Ginger Chicken Congee

Ingredients:
- 1 cup jasmine rice
- 8 cups low-sodium chicken broth
- 2 boneless, skinless chicken breasts
- 2 tbsp fresh ginger, julienned
- 2 cloves garlic, minced
- 1 tbsp soy sauce
- 2 green onions, sliced
- 1 tbsp sesame oil

Instructions:
1. Rinse the rice under cold water until the water runs clear.
2. In a large pot, combine the rice and chicken broth. Bring to a boil over high heat.
3. Once boiling, reduce the heat to low and add the chicken breasts, ginger, and garlic. Simmer for about 1 hour, stirring occasionally, until the rice breaks down and the congee reaches a creamy consistency.
4. Remove the chicken breasts, shred them with a fork, and return the shredded chicken to the pot. Stir in the soy sauce.
5. Serve the congee hot, drizzled with sesame oil and garnished with sliced green onions.

Nutrition Info (per serving):
- Calories: 250
- Protein: 20g
- Carbohydrates: 30g
- Dietary Fiber: 1g
- Sugars: 1g
- Fat: 7g
- Saturated Fat: 1g
- Cholesterol: 45mg
- Sodium: 350mg

Servings: 6

Cooking Time: 1 hour 20 minutes

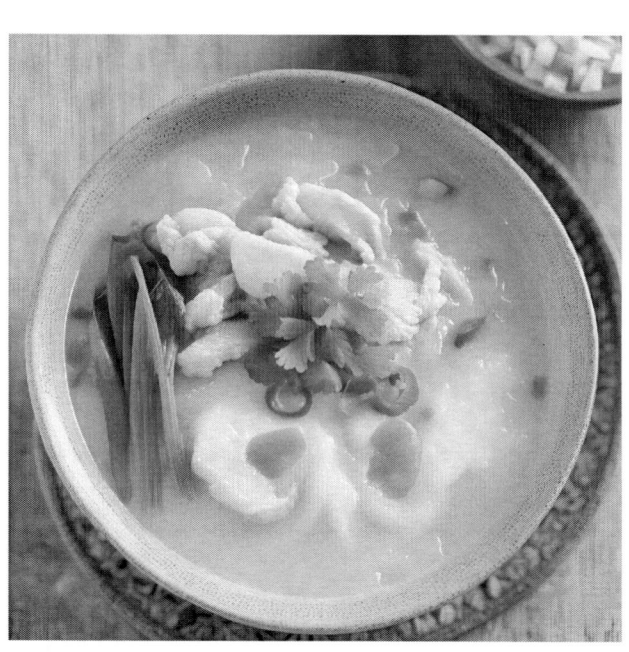

2. Lemon Herb Roasted Chicken

Ingredients:
- 1 whole chicken (about 4 lbs)
- 2 lemons, quartered
- 4 cloves garlic, minced
- 2 tbsp olive oil
- 1 tbsp fresh rosemary, chopped
- 1 tbsp fresh thyme, chopped
- 1 tsp paprika

Instructions:
1. Preheat your oven to 375°F (190°C). Line a roasting pan with foil.
2. In a small bowl, combine the olive oil, minced garlic, chopped rosemary, chopped thyme, and paprika.
3. Rub the olive oil mixture all over the chicken, including under the skin. Stuff the cavity with the lemon quarters.
4. Place the chicken breast-side up in the prepared roasting pan.
5. Roast the chicken for about 1 hour and 30 minutes, or until the internal temperature reaches 165°F (74°C) and the juices run clear.
6. Let the chicken rest for 10 minutes before carving and serving.

Nutrition Info (per serving):
- Calories: 350
- Protein: 28g
- Carbohydrates: 4g
- Dietary Fiber: 1g
- Sugars: 0g
- Fat: 24g
- Saturated Fat: 6g
- Cholesterol: 95mg
- Sodium: 80mg

Servings: 6
Cooking Time: 1 hour 45 minutes

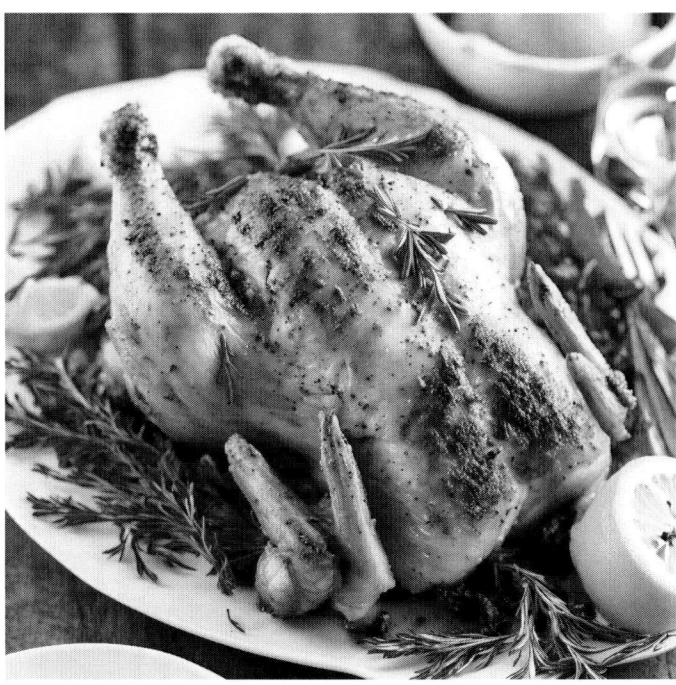

3. Turkey Sweet Potato Skillet

Ingredients:
- 1 lb ground turkey
- 2 medium sweet potatoes, peeled and diced
- 1 red bell pepper, diced
- 1 green bell pepper, diced
- 1 onion, diced
- 2 cloves garlic, minced
- 1 tsp cumin
- 1/2 tsp paprika
- 2 tbsp olive oil
- 1/4 cup fresh cilantro, chopped

Instructions:
1. In a large skillet, heat the olive oil over medium heat. Add the diced sweet potatoes and cook for 8-10 minutes until they start to soften.
2. Add the onion, red bell pepper, green bell pepper, and minced garlic to the skillet. Cook for an additional 5 minutes until the vegetables are tender.
3. Push the vegetables to one side of the skillet and add the ground turkey. Cook until browned, breaking it up with a spoon as it cooks.
4. Stir in the cumin and paprika, mixing everything together. Cook for another 5 minutes until the turkey is fully cooked and the sweet potatoes are tender.
5. Garnish with chopped cilantro before serving.

Nutrition Info (per serving):
- Calories: 320
- Protein: 22g
- Carbohydrates: 28g
- Dietary Fiber: 6g
- Sugars: 7g
- Fat: 15g
- Saturated Fat: 3g
- Cholesterol: 70mg
- Sodium: 80mg

Servings: 4
Cooking Time: 30 minutes

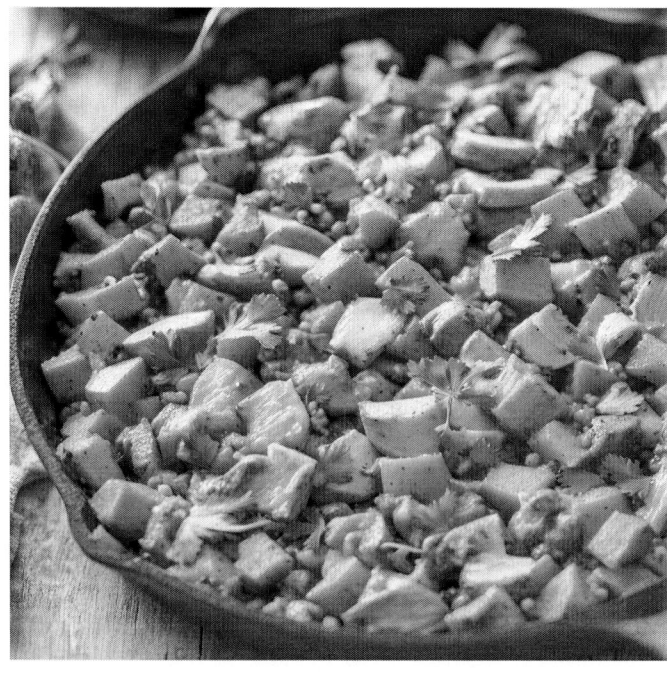

4. Garlic Thyme Chicken Soup

Ingredients:
- 1 lb boneless, skinless chicken thighs
- 8 cups low-sodium chicken broth
- 4 cloves garlic, minced
- 1 onion, diced
- 2 carrots, diced
- 2 celery stalks, diced
- 1 cup pearl barley
- 2 tbsp fresh thyme, chopped
- 1 tbsp olive oil
- 1/4 tsp paprika

Instructions:
1. In a large pot, heat the olive oil over medium heat. Add the minced garlic and diced onion, and cook until the onion is translucent, about 5 minutes.
2. Add the diced carrots and celery to the pot and cook for another 5 minutes until they begin to soften.
3. Pour in the chicken broth and bring to a boil.
4. Add the chicken thighs to the pot. Reduce the heat to low and simmer for 20 minutes.
5. Remove the chicken thighs from the pot and shred them with a fork. Return the shredded chicken to the pot.
6. Stir in the pearl barley, fresh thyme, and paprika. Simmer for an additional 30 minutes until the barley is tender.
7. Serve hot.

Nutrition Info (per serving):
- Calories: 280
- Protein: 24g
- Carbohydrates: 26g
- Dietary Fiber: 5g
- Sugars: 4g
- Fat: 10g
- Saturated Fat: 2g
- Cholesterol: 70mg
- Sodium: 150mg

Servings: 6

Cooking Time: 1 hour

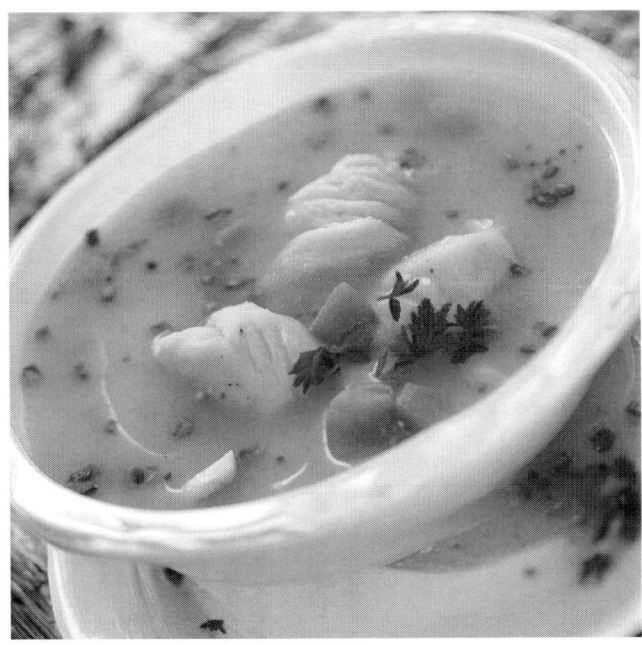

5. Baked Turkey Meatballs with Spinach

Ingredients:
- 1 lb ground turkey
- 1 cup fresh spinach, finely chopped
- 1/2 cup whole wheat bread crumbs
- 1/4 cup grated Parmesan cheese
- 1 egg, beaten
- 2 cloves garlic, minced
- 1 tbsp fresh parsley, chopped
- 1/2 tsp paprika

Instructions:
1. Preheat your oven to 375°F (190°C). Line a baking sheet with parchment paper.
2. In a large bowl, combine the ground turkey, chopped spinach, bread crumbs, Parmesan cheese, beaten egg, minced garlic, parsley, and paprika.
3. Mix until all ingredients are well combined.
4. Form the mixture into small meatballs, about 1 inch in diameter, and place them on the prepared baking sheet.
5. Bake for 20-25 minutes, or until the meatballs are cooked through and lightly browned.
6. Serve warm with your favorite dipping sauce or over whole wheat pasta.

Nutrition Info (per serving):
- Calories: 180
- Protein: 20g
- Carbohydrates: 8g
- Dietary Fiber: 1g
- Sugars: 1g
- Fat: 8g
- Saturated Fat: 2g
- Cholesterol: 70mg
- Sodium: 140mg

Servings: 4
Cooking Time: 30 minutes

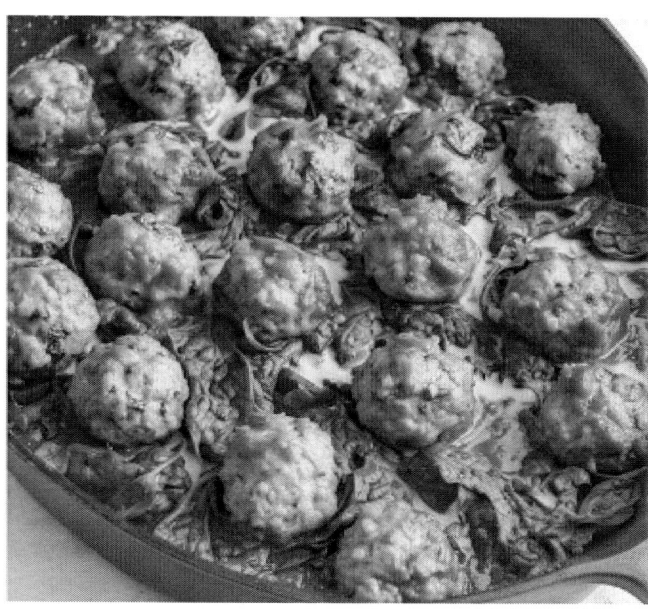

6. Chicken Stew with Soft Vegetables

Ingredients:
- 1 lb boneless, skinless chicken thighs, cut into bite-sized pieces
- 2 cups low-sodium chicken broth
- 2 carrots, sliced
- 2 celery stalks, sliced
- 1 potato, peeled and diced
- 1 onion, chopped
- 2 cloves garlic, minced
- 1 tbsp olive oil
- 1 tsp thyme
- 1/4 tsp paprika

Instructions:
1. Heat the olive oil in a large pot over medium heat. Add the onion and garlic, and cook until the onion is translucent, about 5 minutes.
2. Add the chicken thighs to the pot and cook until browned, about 5 minutes.
3. Add the carrots, celery, and potato to the pot. Pour in the chicken broth and bring to a boil.
4. Reduce the heat to low, add the thyme and paprika, and simmer for 30 minutes, or until the vegetables are tender and the chicken is cooked through.
5. Serve hot.

Nutrition Info (per serving):
- Calories: 250
- Protein: 22g
- Carbohydrates: 18g
- Dietary Fiber: 3g
- Sugars: 4g
- Fat: 10g
- Saturated Fat: 2g
- Cholesterol: 70mg
- Sodium: 150mg

Servings: 4
Cooking Time: 45 minutes

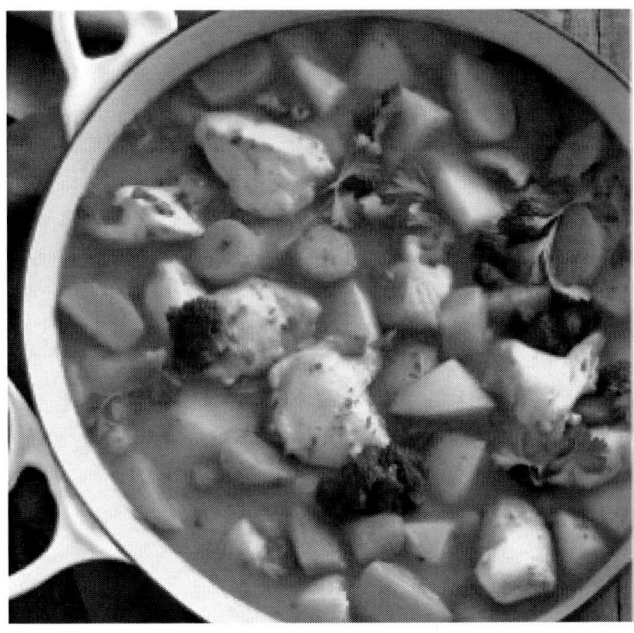

7. Turkey and Zucchini Burgers

Ingredients:
- 1 lb ground turkey
- 1 cup grated zucchini, squeezed dry
- 1/4 cup whole wheat bread crumbs
- 1 egg, beaten
- 2 cloves garlic, minced
- 1 tbsp fresh parsley, chopped
- 1/2 tsp paprika
- 1 tbsp olive oil

Instructions:
1. In a large bowl, combine the ground turkey, grated zucchini, bread crumbs, beaten egg, minced garlic, parsley, and paprika. Mix until well combined.
2. Form the mixture into 4 patties.
3. Heat the olive oil in a large skillet over medium heat. Cook the patties for 5-6 minutes on each side, or until they are cooked through and golden brown.
4. Serve the burgers on whole wheat buns with your favorite toppings.

Nutrition Info (per serving):
- Calories: 210
- Protein: 22g
- Carbohydrates: 7g
- Dietary Fiber: 1g
- Sugars: 1g
- Fat: 10g
- Saturated Fat: 2g
- Cholesterol: 70mg
- Sodium: 130mg

Servings: 4
Cooking Time: 20 minutes

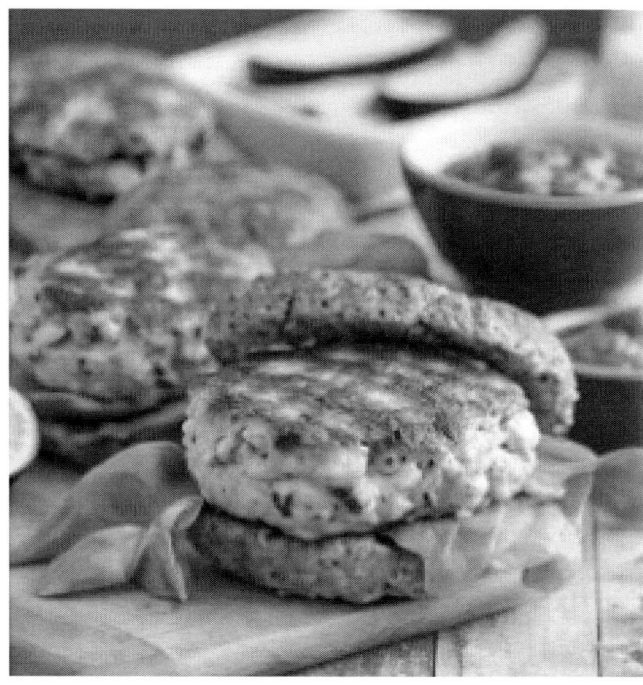

8. Simple Poached Chicken

Ingredients:
- 2 boneless, skinless chicken breasts
- 4 cups low-sodium chicken broth
- 1 small onion, halved
- 2 cloves garlic, smashed
- 1 bay leaf
- 1/4 tsp thyme

Instructions:
1. In a large pot, combine the chicken broth, onion, garlic, bay leaf, and thyme. Bring to a gentle simmer over medium heat.
2. Add the chicken breasts to the pot and reduce the heat to low.
3. Poach the chicken for 15-20 minutes, or until the chicken is cooked through and no longer pink in the center.
4. Remove the chicken from the pot and let it rest for a few minutes before slicing or shredding.
5. Serve the poached chicken with steamed vegetables or over a salad.

Nutrition Info (per serving):
- Calories: 160
- Protein: 30g
- Carbohydrates: 2g
- Dietary Fiber: 0g
- Sugars: 0g
- Fat: 3g
- Saturated Fat: 1g
- Cholesterol: 75mg
- Sodium: 200mg

Servings: 2
Cooking Time: 25 minutes

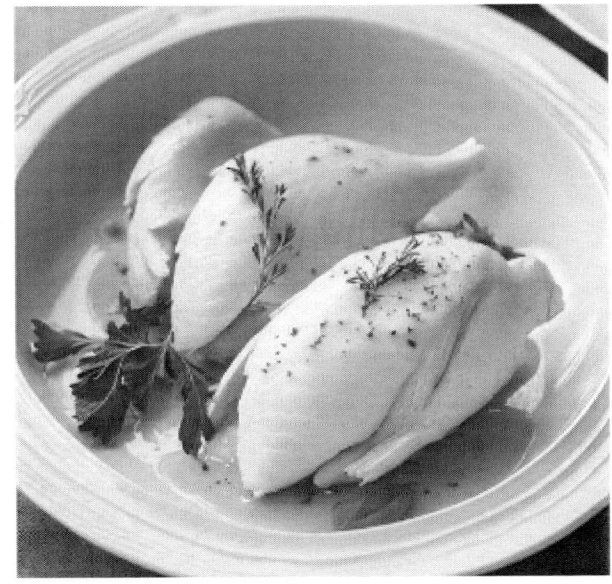

9. Creamy Chicken and Mushroom Soup

Ingredients:
- 1 lb boneless, skinless chicken breasts, diced
- 8 oz mushrooms, sliced
- 1 onion, diced
- 2 cloves garlic, minced
- 4 cups low-sodium chicken broth
- 1 cup low-fat milk
- 1 tbsp olive oil
- 1 tsp thyme
- 1/4 tsp paprika
- 2 tbsp cornstarch mixed with 2 tbsp water

Instructions:
1. Heat the olive oil in a large pot over medium heat. Add the diced onion and minced garlic, and cook until the onion is translucent, about 5 minutes.
2. Add the diced chicken and cook until browned, about 5 minutes.
3. Add the sliced mushrooms and cook for another 5 minutes until they release their juices and become tender.
4. Pour in the chicken broth and bring to a boil. Reduce the heat to low and simmer for 15 minutes.
5. Stir in the milk, thyme, and paprika. Add the cornstarch mixture and cook for another 5 minutes until the soup thickens.
6. Serve hot.

Nutrition Info (per serving):
- Calories: 250
- Protein: 26g
- Carbohydrates: 10g
- Dietary Fiber: 2g
- Sugars: 4g
- Fat: 12g
- Saturated Fat: 2.5g
- Cholesterol: 70mg
- Sodium: 170mg

Servings: 4
Cooking Time: 40 minutes

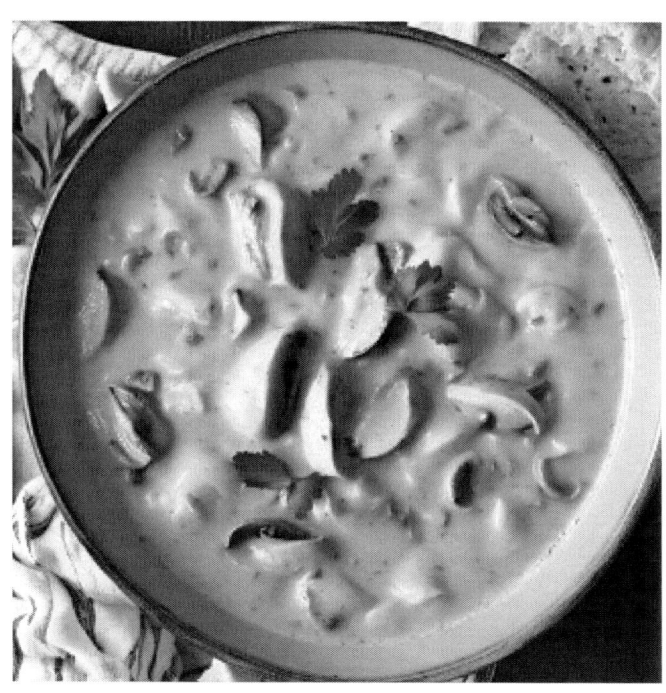

10. Soft Chicken Tacos with Guacamole

Ingredients:
- 1 lb boneless, skinless chicken thighs, diced
- 1 tbsp olive oil
- 1 onion, diced
- 2 cloves garlic, minced
- 1 tsp cumin
- 1/2 tsp paprika
- 8 small whole wheat tortillas
- 1 avocado, mashed
- 1 tbsp lime juice
- 1/4 cup fresh cilantro, chopped

Instructions:
1. In a large skillet, heat the olive oil over medium heat. Add the diced onion and minced garlic, and cook until the onion is translucent, about 5 minutes.
2. Add the diced chicken thighs, cumin, and paprika to the skillet. Cook until the chicken is cooked through and browned, about 10 minutes.
3. While the chicken is cooking, prepare the guacamole by mixing the mashed avocado with lime juice and chopped cilantro.
4. Warm the tortillas in a dry skillet or microwave.
5. Assemble the tacos by placing the chicken mixture on each tortilla and topping with guacamole.
6. Serve immediately.

Nutrition Info (per serving):
- Calories: 300
- Protein: 22g
- Carbohydrates: 20g
- Dietary Fiber: 6g
- Sugars: 2g
- Fat: 15g
- Saturated Fat: 3g
- Cholesterol: 70mg
- Sodium: 180mg

Servings: 4
Cooking Time: 30 minutes

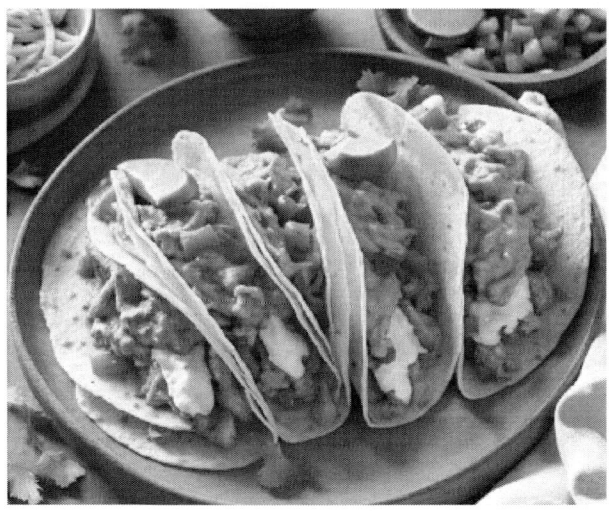

11. Turkey Sloppy Joes

Ingredients:
- 1 lb ground turkey
- 1 onion, diced
- 1 green bell pepper, diced
- 2 cloves garlic, minced
- 1 cup tomato sauce
- 1/4 cup low-sugar ketchup
- 1 tbsp Worcestershire sauce
- 1 tsp paprika
- 4 whole wheat hamburger buns

Instructions:
1. In a large skillet, cook the ground turkey over medium heat until browned, about 5-7 minutes.
2. Add the diced onion, green bell pepper, and minced garlic to the skillet. Cook until the vegetables are tender, about 5 minutes.
3. Stir in the tomato sauce, ketchup, Worcestershire sauce, and paprika. Simmer for 10 minutes, stirring occasionally.
4. Serve the turkey mixture on whole wheat hamburger buns.

Nutrition Info (per serving):
- Calories: 350
- Protein: 25g
- Carbohydrates: 40g
- Dietary Fiber: 6g
- Sugars: 10g
- Fat: 10g
- Saturated Fat: 2g
- Cholesterol: 70mg
- Sodium: 400mg

Servings: 4
Cooking Time: 25 minutes

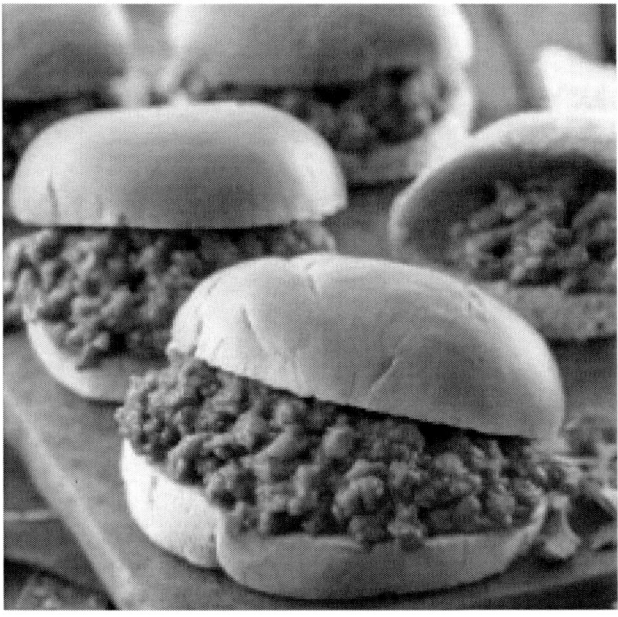

12. Chicken Porridge with Mild Spices
Ingredients:
- 1 cup jasmine rice
- 8 cups low-sodium chicken broth
- 2 boneless, skinless chicken breasts
- 1 onion, finely chopped
- 2 cloves garlic, minced
- 1 tbsp fresh ginger, minced
- 1/2 tsp turmeric
- 1/4 tsp cumin
- 2 green onions, sliced
- 1 tbsp sesame oil

Instructions:
1. Rinse the rice under cold water until the water runs clear.
2. In a large pot, combine the rice and chicken broth. Bring to a boil over high heat.
3. Once boiling, reduce the heat to low and add the chicken breasts, onion, garlic, ginger, turmeric, and cumin. Simmer for about 1 hour, stirring occasionally, until the rice breaks down and the porridge reaches a creamy consistency.
4. Remove the chicken breasts, shred them with a fork, and return the shredded chicken to the pot.
5. Serve the porridge hot, drizzled with sesame oil and garnished with sliced green onions.

Nutrition Info (per serving):
- Calories: 270
- Protein: 22g
- Carbohydrates: 34g
- Dietary Fiber: 1g
- Sugars: 2g
- Fat: 7g
- Saturated Fat: 1g
- Cholesterol: 45mg
- Sodium: 350mg

Servings: 6
Cooking Time: 1 hour 20 minutes

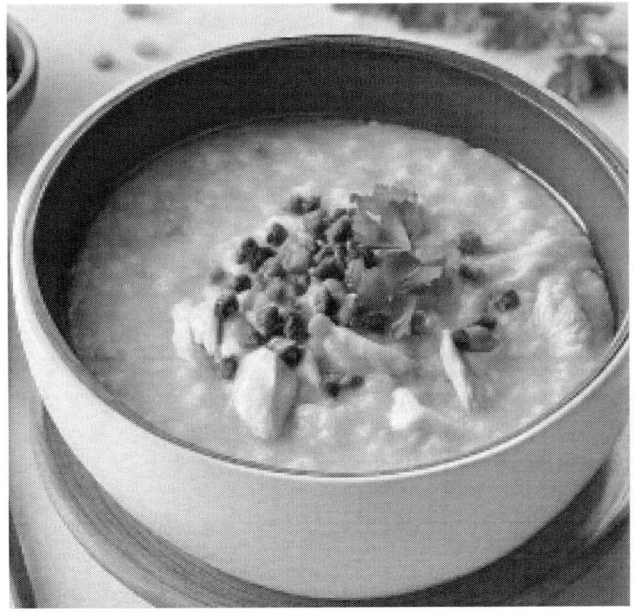

13. Pesto Chicken Pasta with Whole Wheat Noodles

Ingredients:
- 1 lb boneless, skinless chicken breasts, diced
- 8 oz whole wheat pasta
- 1 cup cherry tomatoes, halved
- 1/4 cup prepared pesto
- 2 cloves garlic, minced
- 2 tbsp olive oil
- 1/4 cup grated Parmesan cheese

Instructions:
1. Cook the whole wheat pasta according to the package instructions. Drain and set aside.
2. In a large skillet, heat the olive oil over medium heat. Add the minced garlic and cook for 1-2 minutes until fragrant.
3. Add the diced chicken breasts to the skillet and cook until browned and cooked through, about 5-7 minutes.
4. Stir in the cherry tomatoes and cook for another 2-3 minutes until they start to soften.
5. Add the cooked pasta and pesto to the skillet. Toss to combine and heat through.
6. Serve topped with grated Parmesan cheese.

Nutrition Info (per serving):
- Calories: 400
- Protein: 30g
- Carbohydrates: 42g
- Dietary Fiber: 6g
- Sugars: 4g
- Fat: 14g
- Saturated Fat: 3g
- Cholesterol: 75mg
- Sodium: 220mg

Servings: 4
Cooking Time: 25 minutes

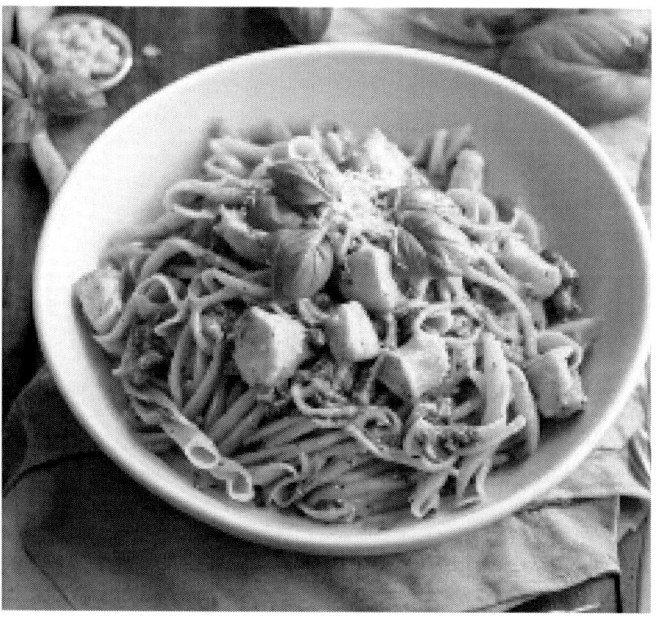

14. Chicken and Broccoli Alfredo

Ingredients:
- 1 lb boneless, skinless chicken breasts, sliced into strips
- 2 cups broccoli florets
- 8 oz whole wheat fettuccine
- 1 cup low-fat milk
- 1/2 cup grated Parmesan cheese
- 2 cloves garlic, minced
- 1 tbsp olive oil
- 1 tbsp cornstarch mixed with 2 tbsp water

Instructions:
1. Cook the whole wheat fettuccine according to the package instructions. Add the broccoli florets to the boiling pasta water during the last 3 minutes of cooking. Drain and set aside.
2. In a large skillet, heat the olive oil over medium heat. Add the minced garlic and cook for 1-2 minutes until fragrant.
3. Add the chicken strips to the skillet and cook until browned and cooked through, about 5-7 minutes.
4. Stir in the low-fat milk and bring to a gentle simmer. Add the cornstarch mixture and cook for another 2-3 minutes until the sauce thickens.
5. Add the cooked pasta and broccoli to the skillet, tossing to coat in the sauce.
6. Stir in the grated Parmesan cheese and serve immediately.

Nutrition Info (per serving):
- Calories: 450
- Protein: 36g
- Carbohydrates: 48g
- Dietary Fiber: 8g
- Sugars: 6g
- Fat: 14g
- Saturated Fat: 4g
- Cholesterol: 80mg
- Sodium: 250mg

Servings: 4
Cooking Time: 30 minutes

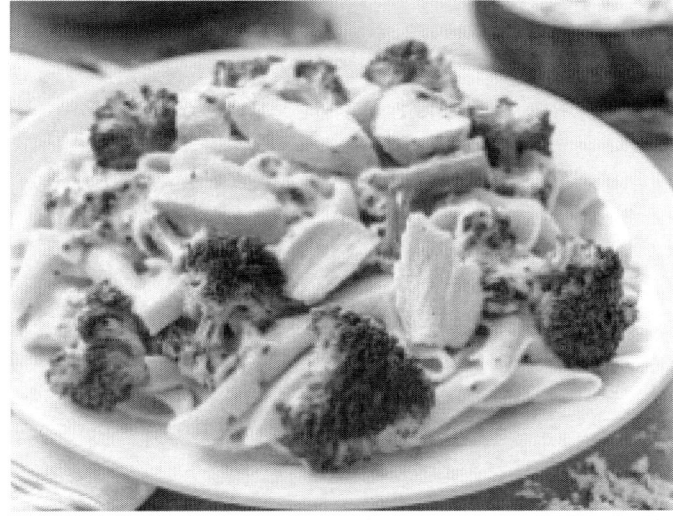

15. Turkey Breast with Sweet Potato Mash

Ingredients:
- 1 lb turkey breast, sliced
- 2 tbsp olive oil
- 2 cloves garlic, minced
- 1 tsp thyme
- 4 medium sweet potatoes, peeled and cubed
- 1/4 cup low-fat milk
- 1 tbsp butter
- 1/4 tsp paprika

Instructions:
1. Preheat your oven to 375°F (190°C). Line a baking sheet with parchment paper.
2. Rub the turkey breast slices with olive oil, minced garlic, and thyme. Place them on the prepared baking sheet.
3. Bake the turkey for 25-30 minutes, or until the internal temperature reaches 165°F (74°C) and the juices run clear.
4. While the turkey is baking, place the cubed sweet potatoes in a large pot of boiling water. Cook until tender, about 15 minutes.
5. Drain the sweet potatoes and return them to the pot. Add the low-fat milk, butter, and paprika. Mash until smooth and creamy.
6. Serve the baked turkey breast slices with the sweet potato mash.

Nutrition Info (per serving):
- Calories: 350
- Protein: 30g
- Carbohydrates: 38g
- Dietary Fiber: 6g
- Sugars: 8g
- Fat: 10g
- Saturated Fat: 3g
- Cholesterol: 70mg
- Sodium: 120mg

Servings: 4
Cooking Time: 40 minutes

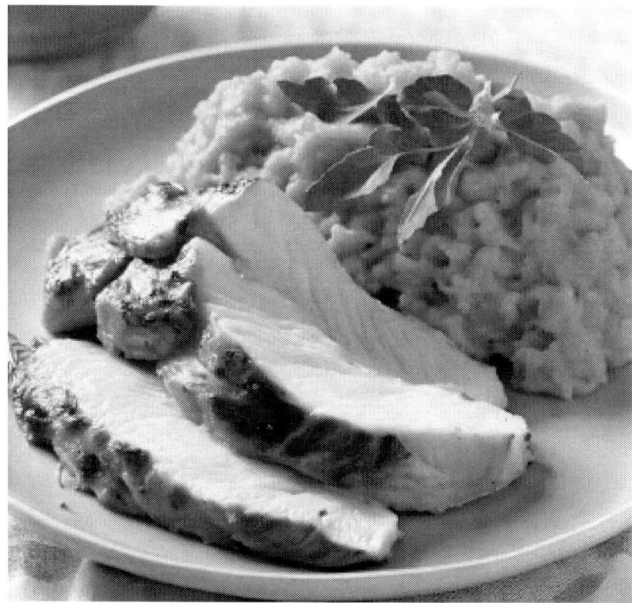

16. Slow-Cooked Chicken with Root Vegetables

Ingredients:
- 4 boneless, skinless chicken thighs
- 2 carrots, sliced
- 2 parsnips, sliced
- 2 potatoes, diced
- 1 onion, chopped
- 3 cloves garlic, minced
- 1 cup low-sodium chicken broth
- 1 tbsp olive oil
- 1 tsp thyme
- 1/4 tsp paprika

Instructions:
1. In a slow cooker, layer the carrots, parsnips, potatoes, onion, and garlic.
2. Place the chicken thighs on top of the vegetables.
3. Drizzle the olive oil over the chicken and sprinkle with thyme and paprika.
4. Pour the chicken broth over everything.
5. Cover and cook on low for 6-7 hours or on high for 3-4 hours, until the chicken and vegetables are tender.
6. Serve hot.

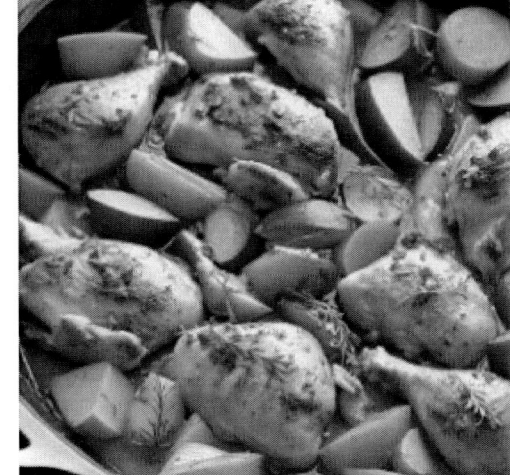

Nutrition Info (per serving):
- Calories: 300
- Protein: 25g
- Carbohydrates: 25g
- Dietary Fiber: 5g
- Sugars: 5g
- Fat: 12g
- Saturated Fat: 3g
- Cholesterol: 90mg
- Sodium: 150mg

Servings: 4
Cooking Time: 6-7 hours on low or 3-4 hours on high

17. Chicken Salad with Greek Yogurt Dressing

Ingredients:
- 2 boneless, skinless chicken breasts, cooked and diced
- 1 cup Greek yogurt
- 1 tbsp Dijon mustard
- 1 tbsp lemon juice
- 1 celery stalk, finely chopped
- 1/4 cup red onion, finely chopped
- 1/4 cup fresh parsley, chopped
- 1/4 tsp paprika

Instructions:
1. In a large bowl, combine the Greek yogurt, Dijon mustard, lemon juice, and paprika. Mix well.
2. Add the diced chicken, celery, red onion, and parsley to the bowl. Toss until the chicken is evenly coated with the dressing.
3. Chill in the refrigerator for at least 30 minutes before serving.
4. Serve on a bed of greens or in a whole wheat pita.

Nutrition Info (per serving):
- Calories: 220
- Protein: 30g
- Carbohydrates: 6g
- Dietary Fiber: 1g
- Sugars: 3g
- Fat: 8g
- Saturated Fat: 2g
- Cholesterol: 75mg
- Sodium: 200mg

Servings: 4

Cooking Time: 15 minutes + 30 minutes chilling

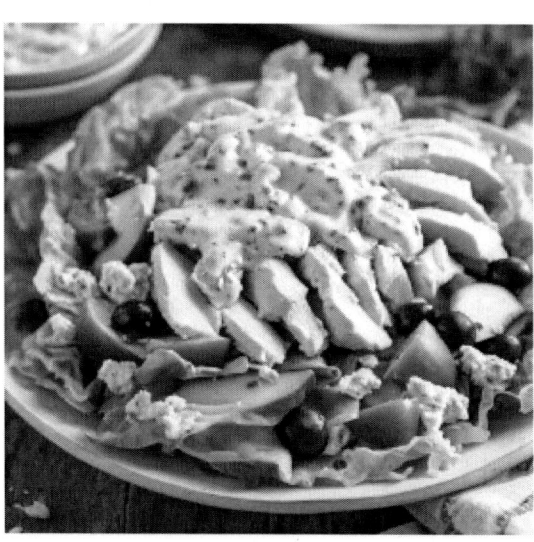

18. Turkey Quinoa Stuffed Peppers

Ingredients:
- 4 large bell peppers, tops cut off and seeds removed
- 1 lb ground turkey
- 1 cup cooked quinoa
- 1 can (14.5 oz) diced tomatoes, drained
- 1 onion, diced
- 2 cloves garlic, minced
- 1 tsp cumin
- 1/2 tsp paprika
- 1/4 cup shredded mozzarella cheese (optional)
- 1 tbsp olive oil

Instructions:
1. Preheat your oven to 375°F (190°C). Line a baking dish with parchment paper.
2. In a large skillet, heat the olive oil over medium heat. Add the diced onion and minced garlic, and cook until the onion is translucent, about 5 minutes.
3. Add the ground turkey to the skillet and cook until browned, about 7-8 minutes.
4. Stir in the cooked quinoa, diced tomatoes, cumin, and paprika. Cook for another 5 minutes until heated through.
5. Stuff each bell pepper with the turkey and quinoa mixture and place them in the prepared baking dish.
6. Top each stuffed pepper with shredded mozzarella cheese, if using.
7. Bake for 25-30 minutes, or until the peppers are tender.
8. Serve hot.

Nutrition Info (per serving):
- Calories: 280
- Protein: 25g
- Carbohydrates: 28g
- Dietary Fiber: 5g
- Sugars: 8g
- Fat: 10g
- Saturated Fat: 3g
- Cholesterol: 70mg
- Sodium: 250mg

Servings: 4
Cooking Time: 45 minutes

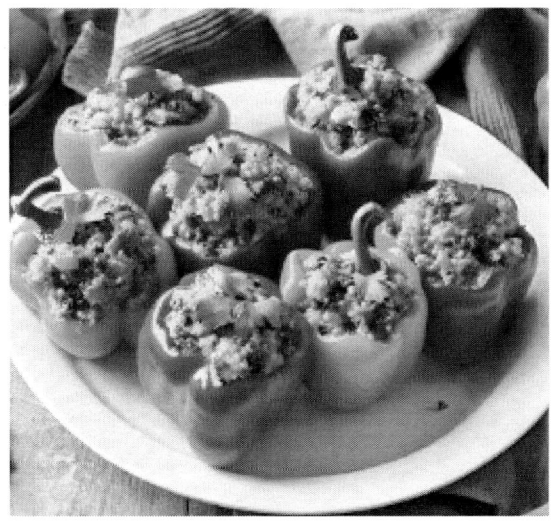

19. Chicken Ginger Noodle Soup

Ingredients:
- 1 lb boneless, skinless chicken breasts, sliced thinly
- 8 cups low-sodium chicken broth
- 1 cup carrots, julienned
- 1 cup snow peas, trimmed
- 1 cup shiitake mushrooms, sliced
- 2 cloves garlic, minced
- 1 tbsp fresh ginger, minced
- 4 oz rice noodles
- 2 tbsp low-sodium soy sauce
- 1 tbsp sesame oil
- 1/4 cup fresh cilantro, chopped

Instructions:
1. In a large pot, heat the sesame oil over medium heat. Add the garlic and ginger, and cook until fragrant, about 2 minutes.
2. Add the chicken broth and bring to a boil.
3. Add the chicken breasts, carrots, snow peas, and shiitake mushrooms. Reduce the heat and simmer for 10 minutes, or until the chicken is cooked through and the vegetables are tender.
4. Stir in the rice noodles and soy sauce, and cook for another 5 minutes until the noodles are tender.
5. Serve hot, garnished with fresh cilantro.

Nutrition Info (per serving):
- Calories: 260
- Protein: 25g
- Carbohydrates: 25g
- Dietary Fiber: 3g
- Sugars: 4g
- Fat: 8g
- Saturated Fat: 1.5g
- Cholesterol: 50mg
- Sodium: 300mg

Servings: 4
Cooking Time: 25 minutes

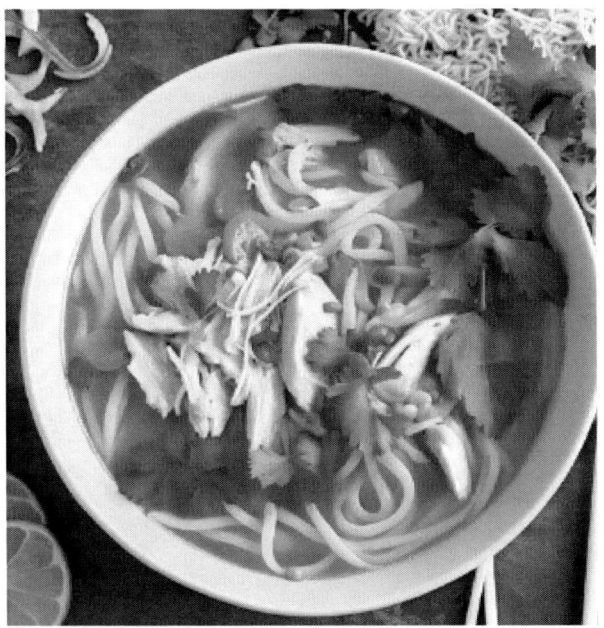

20. Moroccan Spiced Chicken Stew

Ingredients:
- 1 lb boneless, skinless chicken thighs, diced
- 1 onion, diced
- 2 carrots, diced
- 2 potatoes, diced
- 1 can (14.5 oz) diced tomatoes
- 1 cup low-sodium chicken broth
- 1 cup chickpeas, drained and rinsed
- 2 cloves garlic, minced
- 1 tsp cumin
- 1 tsp coriander
- 1 tsp paprika
- 1/2 tsp cinnamon
- 1 tbsp olive oil

Instructions:
1. In a large pot, heat the olive oil over medium heat. Add the diced onion and minced garlic, and cook until the onion is translucent, about 5 minutes.
2. Add the diced chicken thighs and cook until browned, about 5-7 minutes.
3. Stir in the carrots, potatoes, diced tomatoes, chicken broth, chickpeas, cumin, coriander, paprika, and cinnamon.
4. Bring to a boil, then reduce the heat and simmer for 30 minutes, or until the vegetables are tender and the chicken is cooked through.
5. Serve hot.

Nutrition Info (per serving):
- Calories: 300
- Protein: 25g
- Carbohydrates: 30g
- Dietary Fiber: 6g
- Sugars: 7g
- Fat: 10g
- Saturated Fat: 2g
- Cholesterol: 75mg
- Sodium: 280mg

Servings: 4
Cooking Time: 45 minutes

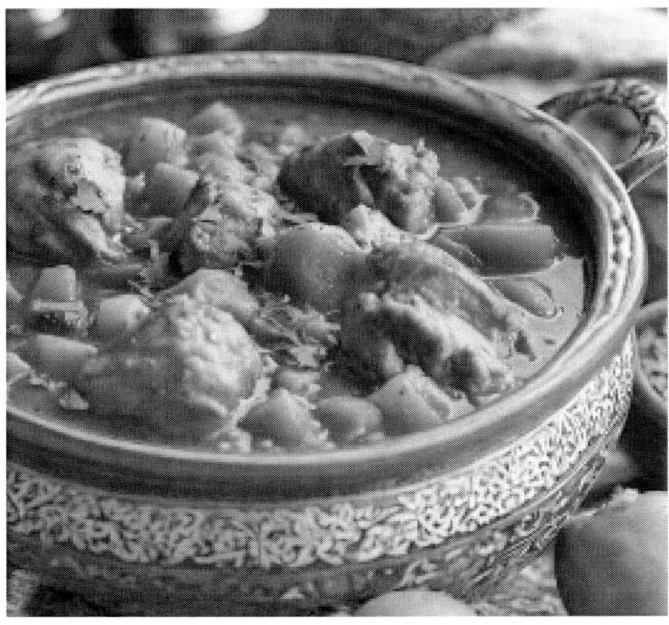

21. Chicken Paillard with Steamed Greens

Ingredients:
- 4 boneless, skinless chicken breasts, pounded thin
- 2 tbsp olive oil
- 1 lemon, juiced
- 2 cloves garlic, minced
- 1 tsp thyme
- 4 cups mixed greens (spinach, kale, chard), steamed
- 1/4 tsp paprika

Instructions:
1. In a large skillet, heat the olive oil over medium-high heat. Add the minced garlic and cook until fragrant, about 1-2 minutes.
2. Add the chicken breasts to the skillet and cook for 3-4 minutes on each side, or until they are golden brown and cooked through.
3. Remove the chicken from the skillet and set aside.
4. In the same skillet, add the lemon juice, thyme, and paprika, stirring to combine.
5. Pour the lemon sauce over the cooked chicken.
6. Serve the chicken paillard with the steamed greens.

Nutrition Info (per serving):
- Calories: 280
- Protein: 30g
- Carbohydrates: 6g
- Dietary Fiber: 3g
- Sugars: 1g
- Fat: 14g
- Saturated Fat: 2.5g
- Cholesterol: 85mg
- Sodium: 120mg

Servings: 4
Cooking Time: 20 minutes

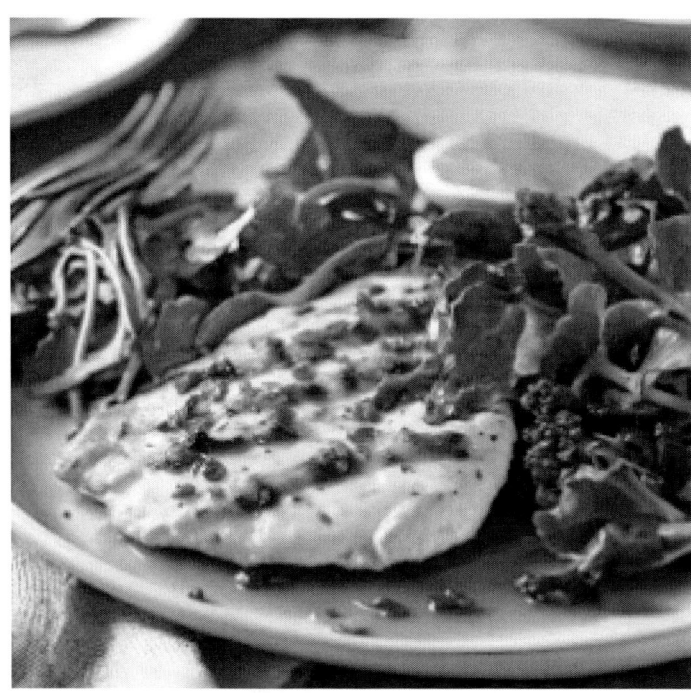

Soup & Stew Recipes

1. Beet and Cabbage Red Soup
Ingredients:
- 2 medium beets, peeled and grated
- 2 cups shredded cabbage
- 1 large carrot, peeled and grated
- 1 onion, diced
- 2 cloves garlic, minced
- 4 cups low-sodium vegetable broth
- 1 can (14.5 oz) diced tomatoes
- 1 tbsp olive oil
- 1 tbsp apple cider vinegar
- 1 tsp caraway seeds
- 1 tsp paprika
- 1/4 cup fresh dill, chopped

Instructions:
1. In a large pot, heat the olive oil over medium heat. Add the diced onion and minced garlic, and cook until the onion is translucent, about 5 minutes.
2. Add the grated beets and carrot to the pot and cook for another 5 minutes, stirring occasionally.
3. Stir in the shredded cabbage, diced tomatoes, vegetable broth, apple cider vinegar, caraway seeds, and paprika.
4. Bring to a boil, then reduce the heat and simmer for 25-30 minutes, or until the vegetables are tender.
5. Serve hot, garnished with fresh dill.

Nutrition Info (per serving):
- Calories: 140
- Protein: 4g
- Carbohydrates: 22g
- Dietary Fiber: 5g
- Sugars: 10g
- Fat: 4g
- Saturated Fat: 0.5g
- Cholesterol: 0mg
- Sodium: 150mg

Servings: 6
Cooking Time: 40 minutes

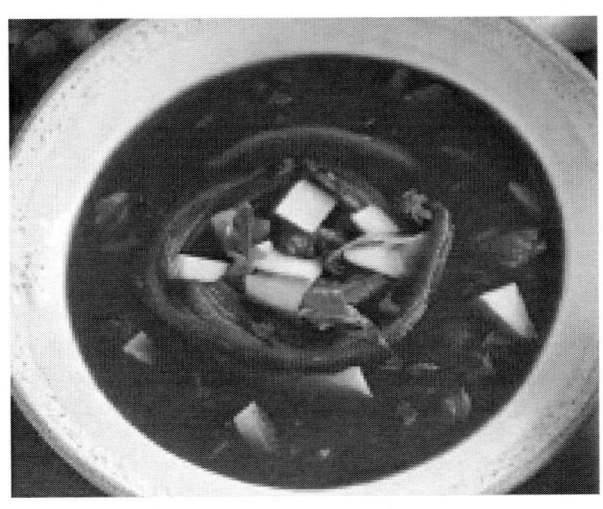

2. Moroccan Lentil Soup

Ingredients:
- 1 cup green or brown lentils, rinsed
- 1 onion, diced
- 2 carrots, diced
- 2 celery stalks, diced
- 2 cloves garlic, minced
- 1 can (14.5 oz) diced tomatoes
- 4 cups low-sodium vegetable broth
- 1 tsp cumin
- 1 tsp coriander
- 1/2 tsp turmeric
- 1/2 tsp cinnamon
- 1 tbsp olive oil
- 1/4 cup fresh cilantro, chopped
- 1 tbsp lemon juice

Instructions:
1. In a large pot, heat the olive oil over medium heat. Add the diced onion, carrots, celery, and minced garlic. Cook until the vegetables are tender, about 5-7 minutes.
2. Stir in the cumin, coriander, turmeric, and cinnamon, and cook for another 1-2 minutes until fragrant.
3. Add the lentils, diced tomatoes, and vegetable broth. Bring to a boil, then reduce the heat and simmer for 25-30 minutes, or until the lentils are tender.
4. Stir in the lemon juice and fresh cilantro before serving.

Nutrition Info (per serving):
- Calories: 200
- Protein: 10g
- Carbohydrates: 30g
- Dietary Fiber: 12g
- Sugars: 6g
- Fat: 5g
- Saturated Fat: 0.5g
- Cholesterol: 0mg
- Sodium: 180mg

Servings: 4
Cooking Time: 40 minutes

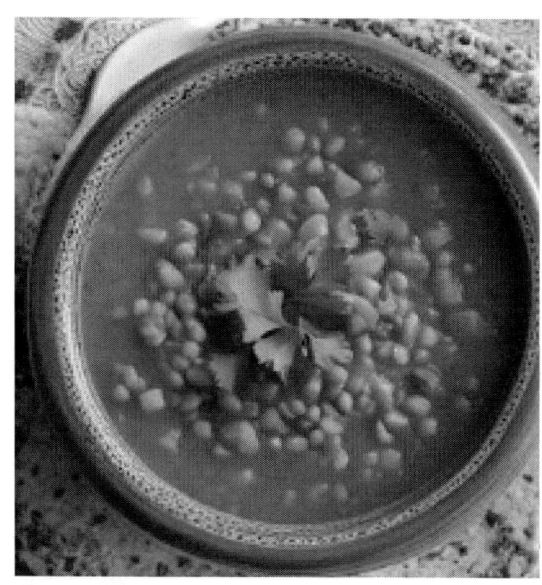

3. Asparagus Soup

Ingredients:
- 2 lbs asparagus, trimmed and cut into 1-inch pieces
- 1 onion, diced
- 2 cloves garlic, minced
- 4 cups low-sodium vegetable broth
- 1 potato, peeled and diced
- 1 tbsp olive oil
- 1/2 tsp thyme
- 1/4 cup plain Greek yogurt (optional for garnish)
- 1 tbsp fresh chives, chopped (optional for garnish)

Instructions:
1. In a large pot, heat the olive oil over medium heat. Add the diced onion and minced garlic, and cook until the onion is translucent, about 5 minutes.
2. Add the asparagus, potato, thyme, and vegetable broth to the pot. Bring to a boil, then reduce the heat and simmer for 20 minutes, or until the vegetables are tender.
3. Use an immersion blender to puree the soup until smooth, or carefully transfer the soup to a blender and puree in batches.
4. Serve hot, garnished with a dollop of Greek yogurt and a sprinkle of fresh chives, if desired.

Nutrition Info (per serving):
- Calories: 130
- Protein: 4g
- Carbohydrates: 19g
- Dietary Fiber: 4g
- Sugars: 4g
- Fat: 5g
- Saturated Fat: 1g
- Cholesterol: 0mg
- Sodium: 160mg

Servings: 4
Cooking Time: 30 minutes

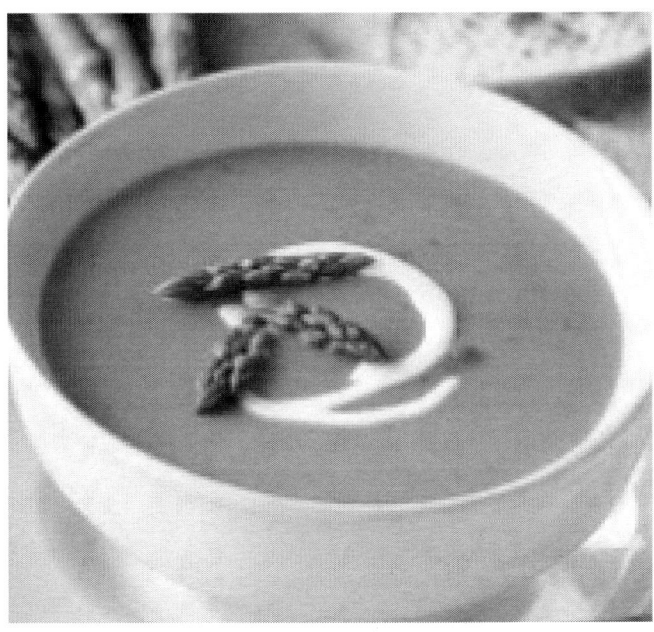

4. Kale and White Bean Soup

Ingredients:
- 1 bunch kale, stems removed and leaves chopped
- 1 can (14.5 oz) white beans, drained and rinsed
- 1 onion, diced
- 2 carrots, diced
- 2 celery stalks, diced
- 2 cloves garlic, minced
- 4 cups low-sodium vegetable broth
- 1 can (14.5 oz) diced tomatoes
- 1 tsp thyme
- 1/2 tsp paprika
- 1 tbsp olive oil
- 1/4 cup fresh parsley, chopped

Instructions:
1. In a large pot, heat the olive oil over medium heat. Add the diced onion, carrots, celery, and minced garlic. Cook until the vegetables are tender, about 5-7 minutes.
2. Stir in the thyme and paprika, and cook for another 1-2 minutes until fragrant.
3. Add the chopped kale, white beans, diced tomatoes, and vegetable broth. Bring to a boil, then reduce the heat and simmer for 20 minutes, or until the kale is tender.
4. Serve hot, garnished with fresh parsley.

Nutrition Info (per serving):
- Calories: 180
- Protein: 7g
- Carbohydrates: 28g
- Dietary Fiber: 8g
- Sugars: 6g
- Fat: 5g
- Saturated Fat: 0.5g
- Cholesterol: 0mg
- Sodium: 180mg

Servings: 4
Cooking Time: 35 minutes

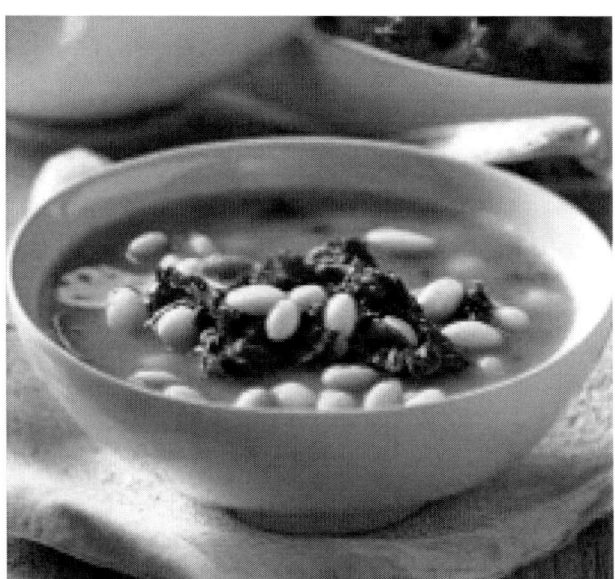

5. Mulligatawny Soup

Ingredients:
- 1 lb boneless, skinless chicken thighs, diced
- 1 onion, diced
- 2 carrots, diced
- 2 celery stalks, diced
- 2 cloves garlic, minced
- 1 apple, peeled and diced
- 1 cup red lentils
- 4 cups low-sodium chicken broth
- 1 can (14.5 oz) diced tomatoes
- 1 can (14 oz) coconut milk
- 1 tbsp olive oil
- 1 tbsp curry powder
- 1 tsp turmeric
- 1/4 tsp cumin
- 1/4 cup fresh cilantro, chopped (optional for garnish)

Instructions:
1. In a large pot, heat the olive oil over medium heat. Add the diced onion, carrots, celery, and minced garlic. Cook until the vegetables are tender, about 5-7 minutes.
2. Add the diced chicken thighs and cook until browned, about 5-7 minutes.
3. Stir in the curry powder, turmeric, and cumin, and cook for another 1-2 minutes until fragrant.
4. Add the diced apple, red lentils, chicken broth, diced tomatoes, and coconut milk. Bring to a boil, then reduce the heat and simmer for 25-30 minutes, or until the lentils and vegetables are tender.
5. Serve hot, garnished with fresh cilantro, if desired.

Nutrition Info (per serving):
- Calories: 320
- Protein: 25g
- Carbohydrates: 30g
- Dietary Fiber: 8g
- Sugars: 8g
- Fat: 12g
- Saturated Fat: 6g
- Cholesterol: 55mg
- Sodium: 220mg

Servings: 6
Cooking Time: 45 minutes

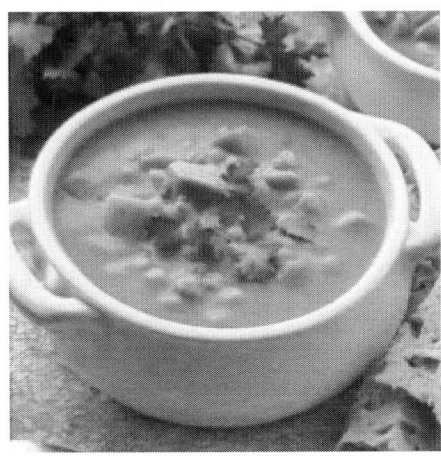

6. French Onion Soup

Ingredients:
- 4 large onions, thinly sliced
- 2 cloves garlic, minced
- 4 cups low-sodium beef broth
- 2 cups low-sodium chicken broth
- 1/2 cup dry white wine
- 1 tbsp olive oil
- 1 tbsp balsamic vinegar
- 1 tsp thyme
- 4 slices whole grain baguette, toasted
- 1/2 cup grated Gruyère cheese

Instructions:
1. In a large pot, heat the olive oil over medium heat. Add the sliced onions and cook, stirring frequently, until they are caramelized, about 25-30 minutes.
2. Add the minced garlic and cook for another 1-2 minutes.
3. Stir in the balsamic vinegar and thyme.
4. Pour in the beef broth, chicken broth, and white wine. Bring to a boil, then reduce the heat and simmer for 20 minutes.
5. Preheat the broiler.
6. Ladle the soup into oven-safe bowls. Top each with a slice of toasted baguette and a sprinkle of Gruyère cheese.
7. Place the bowls under the broiler until the cheese is melted and bubbly, about 2-3 minutes.
8. Serve hot.

Nutrition Info (per serving):
- Calories: 280
- Protein: 10g
- Carbohydrates: 35g
- Dietary Fiber: 4g
- Sugars: 10g
- Fat: 10g
- Saturated Fat: 3g
- Cholesterol: 20mg
- Sodium: 350mg

Servings: 4
Cooking Time: 1 hour

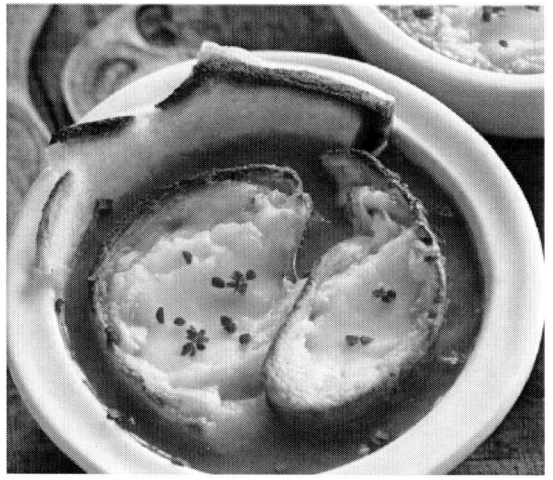

7. Spiced Pumpkin and Carrot Stew

Ingredients:
- 1 lb pumpkin, peeled and cubed
- 2 large carrots, peeled and sliced
- 1 onion, diced
- 2 cloves garlic, minced
- 4 cups low-sodium vegetable broth
- 1 can (14.5 oz) diced tomatoes
- 1 can (14 oz) coconut milk
- 1 tbsp olive oil
- 1 tsp cumin
- 1 tsp coriander
- 1/2 tsp cinnamon
- 1/4 tsp nutmeg
- 1/4 cup fresh cilantro, chopped (optional for garnish)

Instructions:
1. In a large pot, heat the olive oil over medium heat. Add the diced onion and minced garlic, and cook until the onion is translucent, about 5 minutes.
2. Stir in the cumin, coriander, cinnamon, and nutmeg, and cook for another 1-2 minutes until fragrant.
3. Add the cubed pumpkin, sliced carrots, vegetable broth, diced tomatoes, and coconut milk. Bring to a boil, then reduce the heat and simmer for 25-30 minutes, or until the vegetables are tender.
4. Serve hot, garnished with fresh cilantro, if desired.

Nutrition Info (per serving):
- Calories: 220
- Protein: 4g
- Carbohydrates: 25g
- Dietary Fiber: 6g
- Sugars: 10g
- Fat: 12g
- Saturated Fat: 8g
- Cholesterol: 0mg
- Sodium: 250mg

Servings: 6

Cooking Time: 40 minutes

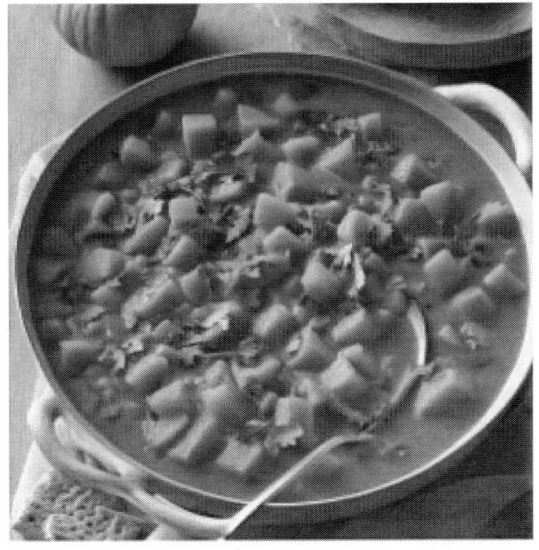

8. Potato Leek Soup

Ingredients:
- 4 large leeks, white and light green parts only, sliced
- 4 medium potatoes, peeled and diced
- 1 onion, diced
- 2 cloves garlic, minced
- 4 cups low-sodium vegetable broth
- 1 cup low-fat milk
- 1 tbsp olive oil
- 1 tsp thyme
- 1/4 tsp paprika

Instructions:
1. In a large pot, heat the olive oil over medium heat. Add the sliced leeks, diced onion, and minced garlic. Cook until the vegetables are tender, about 5-7 minutes.
2. Add the diced potatoes, vegetable broth, thyme, and paprika. Bring to a boil, then reduce the heat and simmer for 20 minutes, or until the potatoes are tender.
3. Use an immersion blender to puree the soup until smooth, or carefully transfer the soup to a blender and puree in batches.
4. Stir in the low-fat milk and heat through.
5. Serve hot.

Nutrition Info (per serving):
- Calories: 180
- Protein: 4g
- Carbohydrates: 30g
- Dietary Fiber: 4g
- Sugars: 6g
- Fat: 5g
- Saturated Fat: 1g
- Cholesterol: 0mg
- Sodium: 150mg

Servings: 6
Cooking Time: 30 minutes

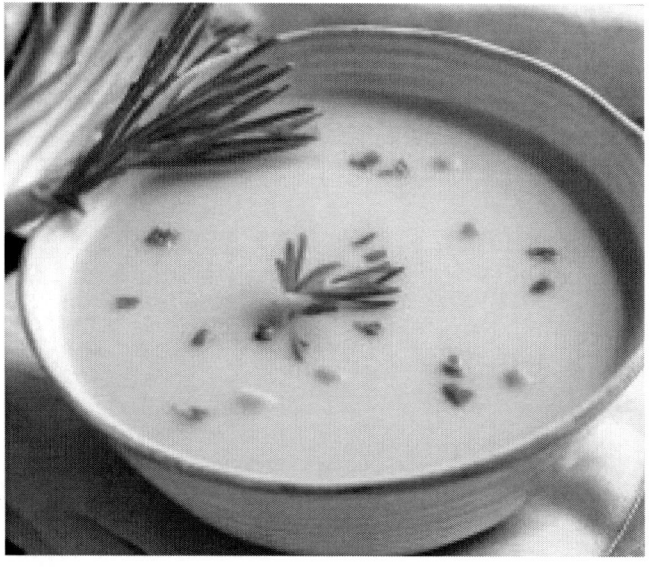

9. Corn Chowder

Ingredients:
- 4 cups corn kernels (fresh or frozen)
- 2 potatoes, peeled and diced
- 1 onion, diced
- 2 cloves garlic, minced
- 4 cups low-sodium vegetable broth
- 1 cup low-fat milk
- 1 red bell pepper, diced
- 2 celery stalks, diced
- 1 tbsp olive oil
- 1 tsp thyme
- 1/4 tsp paprika

Instructions:
1. In a large pot, heat the olive oil over medium heat. Add the diced onion, red bell pepper, celery, and minced garlic. Cook until the vegetables are tender, about 5-7 minutes.
2. Add the corn kernels, diced potatoes, vegetable broth, thyme, and paprika. Bring to a boil, then reduce the heat and simmer for 20 minutes, or until the potatoes are tender.
3. Use an immersion blender to partially puree the soup, leaving some chunks for texture, or carefully transfer half the soup to a blender and puree, then return it to the pot.
4. Stir in the low-fat milk and heat through.
5. Serve hot.

Nutrition Info (per serving):
- Calories: 200
- Protein: 5g
- Carbohydrates: 36g
- Dietary Fiber: 6g
- Sugars: 9g
- Fat: 5g
- Saturated Fat: 1g
- Cholesterol: 0mg
- Sodium: 150mg

Servings: 6
Cooking Time: 30 minutes

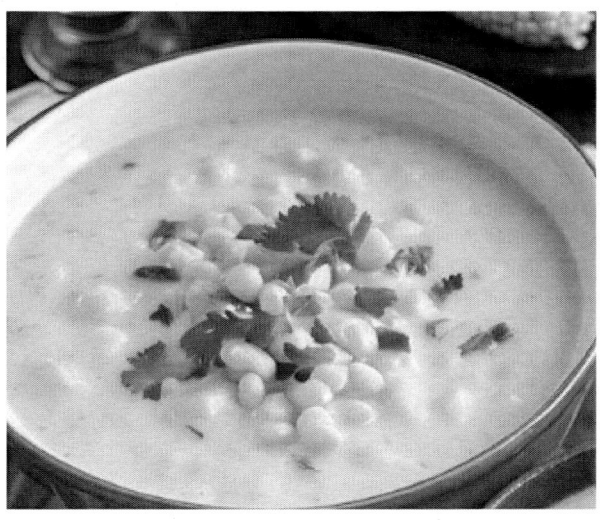

10. Cabbage Soup

Ingredients:
- 1 small head of cabbage, chopped
- 2 carrots, sliced
- 2 celery stalks, sliced
- 1 onion, diced
- 2 cloves garlic, minced
- 4 cups low-sodium vegetable broth
- 1 can (14.5 oz) diced tomatoes
- 1 tbsp olive oil
- 1 tsp thyme
- 1/2 tsp paprika

Instructions:
1. In a large pot, heat the olive oil over medium heat. Add the diced onion and minced garlic, and cook until the onion is translucent, about 5 minutes.
2. Add the sliced carrots and celery, and cook for another 5 minutes until they start to soften.
3. Stir in the chopped cabbage, diced tomatoes, vegetable broth, thyme, and paprika. Bring to a boil, then reduce the heat and simmer for 25-30 minutes, or until the vegetables are tender.
4. Serve hot.

Nutrition Info (per serving):
- Calories: 120
- Protein: 4g
- Carbohydrates: 24g
- Dietary Fiber: 7g
- Sugars: 10g
- Fat: 3g
- Saturated Fat: 0.5g
- Cholesterol: 0mg
- Sodium: 150mg

Servings: 6
Cooking Time: 40 minutes

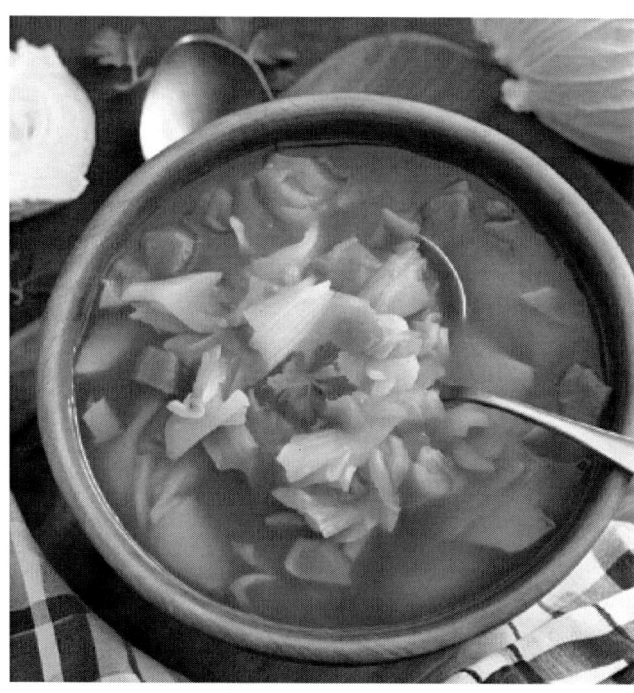

11. Cauliflower and Leek Soup

Ingredients:
- 1 large head of cauliflower, chopped
- 2 large leeks, white and light green parts only, sliced
- 1 onion, diced
- 2 cloves garlic, minced
- 4 cups low-sodium vegetable broth
- 1 cup low-fat milk
- 1 tbsp olive oil
- 1/2 tsp thyme
- 1/4 tsp paprika

Instructions:
1. In a large pot, heat the olive oil over medium heat. Add the sliced leeks, diced onion, and minced garlic. Cook until the vegetables are tender, about 5-7 minutes.
2. Add the chopped cauliflower, vegetable broth, thyme, and paprika. Bring to a boil, then reduce the heat and simmer for 20 minutes, or until the cauliflower is tender.
3. Use an immersion blender to puree the soup until smooth, or carefully transfer the soup to a blender and puree in batches.
4. Stir in the low-fat milk and heat through.
5. Serve hot.

Nutrition Info (per serving):
- Calories: 130
- Protein: 4g
- Carbohydrates: 20g
- Dietary Fiber: 5g
- Sugars: 6g
- Fat: 5g
- Saturated Fat: 1g
- Cholesterol: 0mg
- Sodium: 160mg

Servings: 6
Cooking Time: 30 minutes

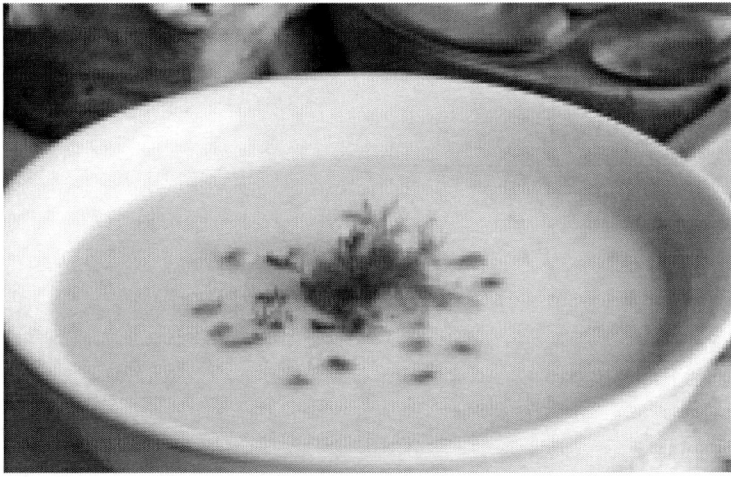

12. Oxtail Stew

Ingredients:
- 2 lbs oxtails
- 1 onion, diced
- 2 carrots, diced
- 2 celery stalks, diced
- 4 cloves garlic, minced
- 1 can (14.5 oz) diced tomatoes
- 4 cups low-sodium beef broth
- 1 cup red wine (optional, can substitute with more broth)
- 2 tbsp olive oil
- 1 tsp thyme
- 1 bay leaf
- 1/4 tsp paprika

Instructions:
1. In a large pot, heat the olive oil over medium-high heat. Add the oxtails and brown on all sides, about 5-7 minutes.
2. Remove the oxtails from the pot and set aside. Add the diced onion, carrots, celery, and minced garlic to the pot. Cook until the vegetables are tender, about 5-7 minutes.
3. Stir in the diced tomatoes, beef broth, red wine (if using), thyme, bay leaf, and paprika. Return the oxtails to the pot.
4. Bring to a boil, then reduce the heat and simmer for 2-3 hours, or until the oxtails are tender and the meat is falling off the bone.
5. Remove the bay leaf before serving.
6. Serve hot.

Nutrition Info (per serving):
- Calories: 350
- Protein: 25g
- Carbohydrates: 15g
- Dietary Fiber: 3g
- Sugars: 6g
- Fat: 20g
- Saturated Fat: 8g
- Cholesterol: 90mg
- Sodium: 300mg

Servings: 6
Cooking Time: 2-3 hours

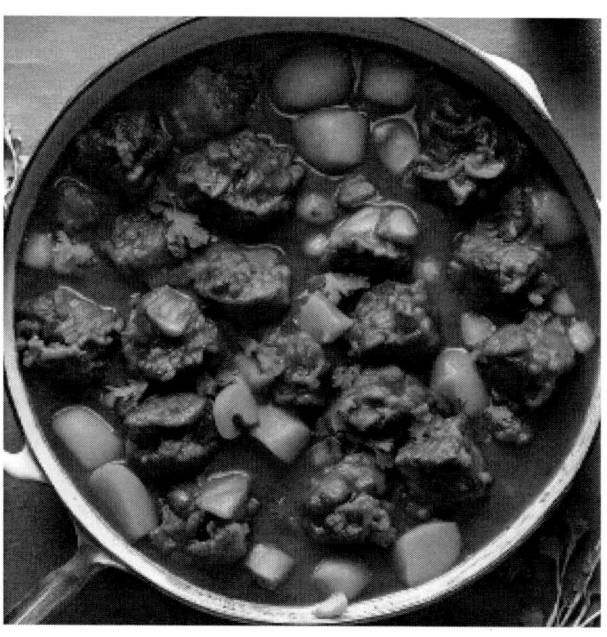

13. Zucchini Basil Soup

Ingredients:
- 4 medium zucchinis, chopped
- 1 onion, diced
- 2 cloves garlic, minced
- 4 cups low-sodium vegetable broth
- 1 cup fresh basil leaves
- 1/2 cup low-fat Greek yogurt
- 1 tbsp olive oil
- 1/2 tsp thyme

Instructions:
1. In a large pot, heat the olive oil over medium heat. Add the diced onion and minced garlic. Cook until the onion is translucent, about 5 minutes.
2. Add the chopped zucchinis and thyme. Cook for another 5 minutes.
3. Pour in the vegetable broth and bring to a boil. Reduce the heat and simmer for 20 minutes, or until the zucchini is tender.
4. Stir in the fresh basil leaves.
5. Use an immersion blender to puree the soup until smooth, or carefully transfer the soup to a blender and puree in batches.
6. Stir in the Greek yogurt until well combined.
7. Serve hot.

Nutrition Info (per serving):
- Calories: 110
- Protein: 5g
- Carbohydrates: 15g
- Dietary Fiber: 3g
- Sugars: 7g
- Fat: 4g
- Saturated Fat: 1g
- Cholesterol: 5mg
- Sodium: 150mg

Servings: 6
Cooking Time: 30 minutes

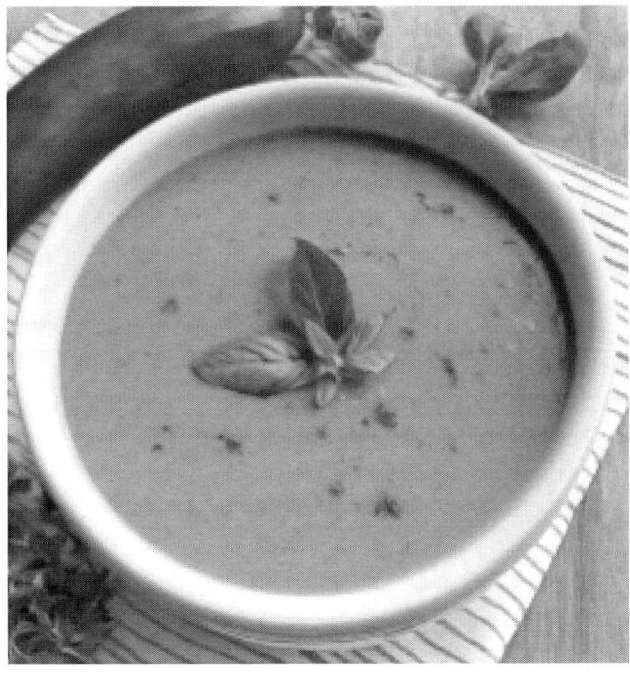

14. Italian Wedding Soup

Ingredients:
- 1/2 lb ground turkey
- 1/2 cup whole wheat bread crumbs
- 1/4 cup grated Parmesan cheese
- 1 egg, beaten
- 1 tsp garlic powder
- 1 tsp thyme
- 4 cups low-sodium chicken broth
- 1 onion, diced
- 2 carrots, diced
- 2 celery stalks, diced
- 1 cup acini di pepe or other small pasta
- 4 cups fresh spinach, chopped
- 1 tbsp olive oil

Instructions:
1. In a bowl, combine the ground turkey, bread crumbs, Parmesan cheese, beaten egg, garlic powder, and half of the thyme. Mix well and form into small meatballs.
2. In a large pot, heat the olive oil over medium heat. Add the meatballs and cook until browned on all sides, about 5-7 minutes. Remove the meatballs from the pot and set aside.
3. Add the diced onion, carrots, and celery to the pot. Cook until the vegetables are tender, about 5-7 minutes.
4. Pour in the chicken broth and bring to a boil. Add the meatballs back to the pot along with the remaining thyme.
5. Stir in the acini di pepe pasta and cook for 10 minutes, or until the pasta is tender.
6. Add the chopped spinach and cook for another 2-3 minutes until wilted.
7. Serve hot.

Nutrition Info (per serving):
- Calories: 250
- Protein: 18g
- Carbohydrates: 25g
- Dietary Fiber: 4g
- Sugars: 6g
- Fat: 10g
- Saturated Fat: 3g
- Cholesterol: 70mg
- Sodium: 250mg

Servings: 6
Cooking Time: 40 minutes

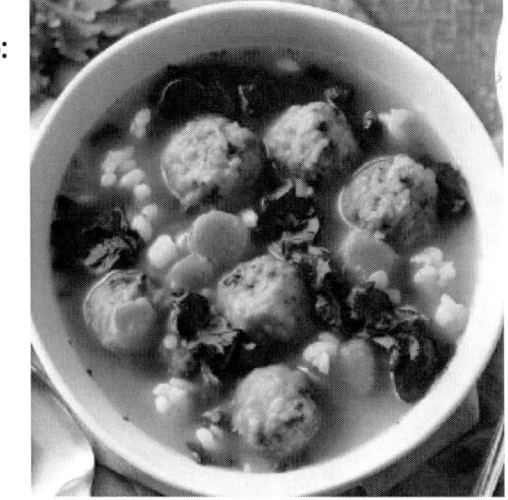

15. Broccoli and Cheese Soup

Ingredients:
- 4 cups broccoli florets
- 1 onion, diced
- 2 cloves garlic, minced
- 4 cups low-sodium vegetable broth
- 1 cup low-fat milk
- 1 cup shredded cheddar cheese
- 1 tbsp olive oil
- 1/2 tsp thyme
- 1/4 tsp paprika

Instructions:
1. In a large pot, heat the olive oil over medium heat. Add the diced onion and minced garlic. Cook until the onion is translucent, about 5 minutes.
2. Add the broccoli florets, thyme, and vegetable broth. Bring to a boil, then reduce the heat and simmer for 15 minutes, or until the broccoli is tender.
3. Use an immersion blender to puree the soup until smooth, or carefully transfer the soup to a blender and puree in batches.
4. Stir in the low-fat milk and shredded cheddar cheese until the cheese is melted and well combined.
5. Serve hot.

Nutrition Info (per serving):
- Calories: 200
- Protein: 10g
- Carbohydrates: 20g
- Dietary Fiber: 4g
- Sugars: 6g
- Fat: 10g
- Saturated Fat: 4g
- Cholesterol: 25mg
- Sodium: 200mg

Servings: 6
Cooking Time: 30 minutes

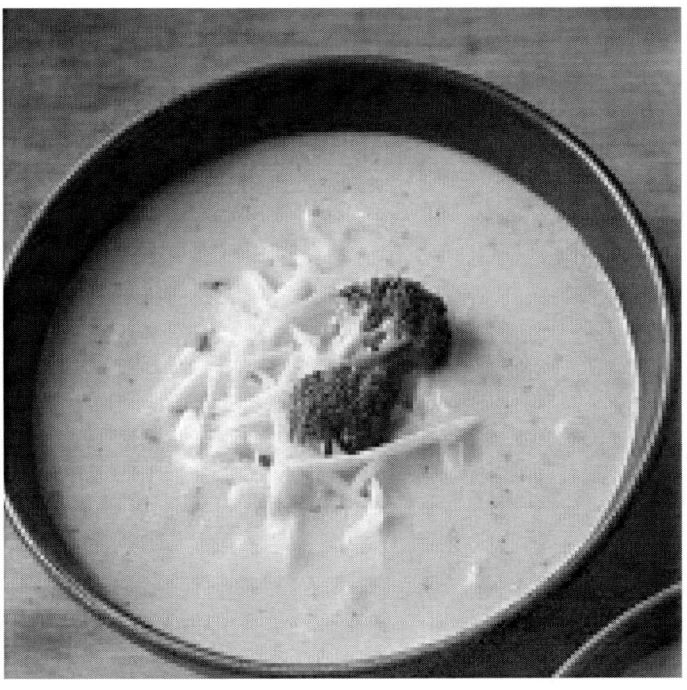

16. Vegetable Beef Soup

Ingredients:
- 1 lb beef stew meat, cut into bite-sized pieces
- 1 onion, diced
- 2 carrots, sliced
- 2 celery stalks, sliced
- 2 potatoes, diced
- 1 cup green beans, trimmed and cut into 1-inch pieces
- 1 can (14.5 oz) diced tomatoes
- 4 cups low-sodium beef broth
- 1 tbsp olive oil
- 1 tsp thyme
- 1/2 tsp paprika
- 1 bay leaf

Instructions:
1. In a large pot, heat the olive oil over medium heat. Add the beef stew meat and cook until browned on all sides, about 5-7 minutes.
2. Add the diced onion, carrots, and celery to the pot. Cook until the vegetables are tender, about 5-7 minutes.
3. Stir in the diced tomatoes, beef broth, thyme, paprika, and bay leaf. Bring to a boil.
4. Add the diced potatoes and green beans. Reduce the heat and simmer for 30 minutes, or until the vegetables and beef are tender.
5. Remove the bay leaf before serving.
6. Serve hot.

Nutrition Info (per serving):
- Calories: 250
- Protein: 22g
- Carbohydrates: 20g
- Dietary Fiber: 4g
- Sugars: 5g
- Fat: 10g
- Saturated Fat: 3g
- Cholesterol: 50mg
- Sodium: 250mg

Servings: 6
Cooking Time: 45 minutes

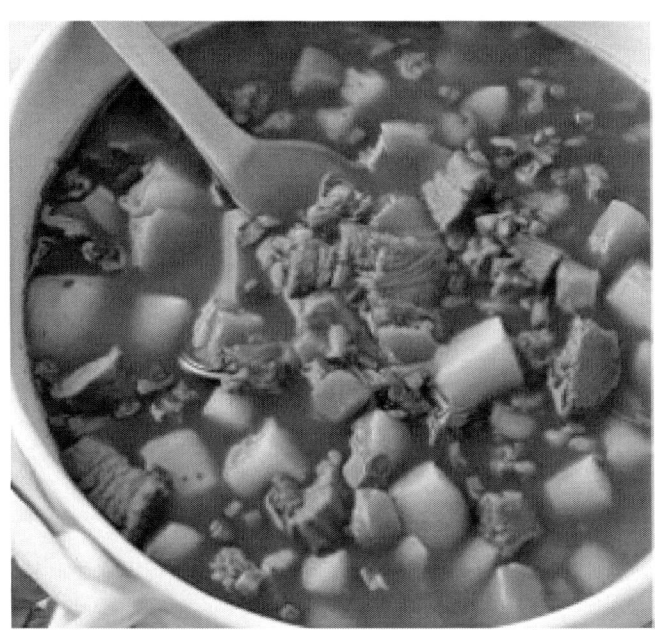

17. Split Pea and Ham Soup

Ingredients:
- 1 lb dried split peas, rinsed
- 1 lb ham, diced
- 1 onion, diced
- 2 carrots, sliced
- 2 celery stalks, sliced
- 2 cloves garlic, minced
- 6 cups low-sodium chicken broth
- 1 tbsp olive oil
- 1 tsp thyme
- 1/2 tsp paprika

Instructions:
1. In a large pot, heat the olive oil over medium heat. Add the diced onion, carrots, celery, and minced garlic. Cook until the vegetables are tender, about 5-7 minutes.
2. Add the diced ham and cook for another 3-4 minutes.
3. Stir in the split peas, chicken broth, thyme, and paprika. Bring to a boil.
4. Reduce the heat and simmer for 1 hour, or until the split peas are tender.
5. Serve hot.

Nutrition Info (per serving):
- Calories: 280
- Protein: 22g
- Carbohydrates: 35g
- Dietary Fiber: 13g
- Sugars: 6g
- Fat: 6g
- Saturated Fat: 2g
- Cholesterol: 35mg
- Sodium: 300mg

Servings: 6

Cooking Time: 1 hour 15 minutes

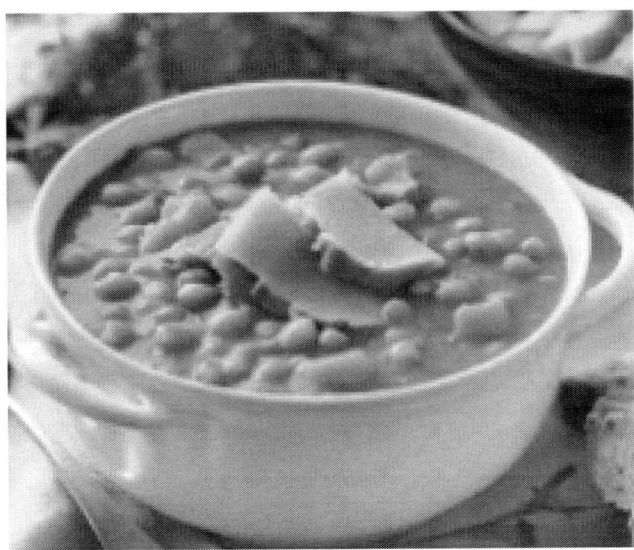

18. Thai Coconut Chicken Soup

Ingredients:
- 1 lb boneless, skinless chicken breasts, sliced thinly
- 1 can (14 oz) coconut milk
- 4 cups low-sodium chicken broth
- 1 cup sliced mushrooms
- 1 red bell pepper, sliced
- 2 cloves garlic, minced
- 1 tbsp fresh ginger, minced
- 2 tbsp fish sauce
- 1 tbsp olive oil
- 1 tbsp lime juice
- 1/4 cup fresh cilantro, chopped (optional for garnish)

Instructions:
1. In a large pot, heat the olive oil over medium heat. Add the minced garlic and ginger, and cook until fragrant, about 1-2 minutes.
2. Add the sliced mushrooms and red bell pepper. Cook for another 3-4 minutes.
3. Pour in the coconut milk and chicken broth. Bring to a boil.
4. Add the sliced chicken breasts and fish sauce. Reduce the heat and simmer for 10-15 minutes, or until the chicken is cooked through.
5. Stir in the lime juice.
6. Serve hot, garnished with fresh cilantro, if desired.

Nutrition Info (per serving):
- Calories: 300
- Protein: 22g
- Carbohydrates: 10g
- Dietary Fiber: 2g
- Sugars: 4g
- Fat: 20g
- Saturated Fat: 14g
- Cholesterol: 55mg
- Sodium: 350mg

Servings: 4
Cooking Time: 30 minutes

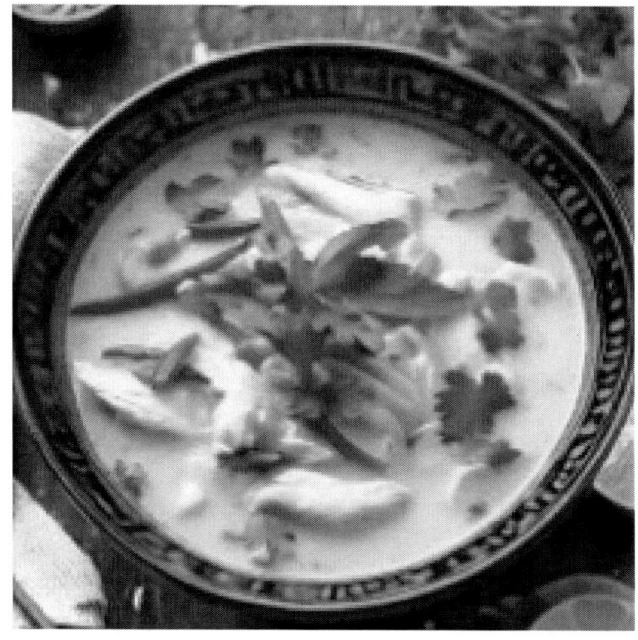

19. Lentil and Carrot Soup

Ingredients:
- 1 cup dried lentils, rinsed
- 4 large carrots, sliced
- 1 onion, diced
- 2 cloves garlic, minced
- 4 cups low-sodium vegetable broth
- 1 can (14.5 oz) diced tomatoes
- 1 tbsp olive oil
- 1 tsp cumin
- 1/2 tsp coriander
- 1/4 tsp paprika

Instructions:
1. In a large pot, heat the olive oil over medium heat. Add the diced onion, carrots, and minced garlic. Cook until the vegetables are tender, about 5-7 minutes.
2. Stir in the cumin, coriander, and paprika, and cook for another 1-2 minutes until fragrant.
3. Add the lentils, vegetable broth, and diced tomatoes. Bring to a boil.
4. Reduce the heat and simmer for 25-30 minutes, or until the lentils are tender.
5. Serve hot.

Nutrition Info (per serving):
- Calories: 200
- Protein: 10g
- Carbohydrates: 35g
- Dietary Fiber: 10g
- Sugars: 9g
- Fat: 4g
- Saturated Fat: 0.5g
- Cholesterol: 0mg
- Sodium: 200mg

Servings: 4
Cooking Time: 35 minutes

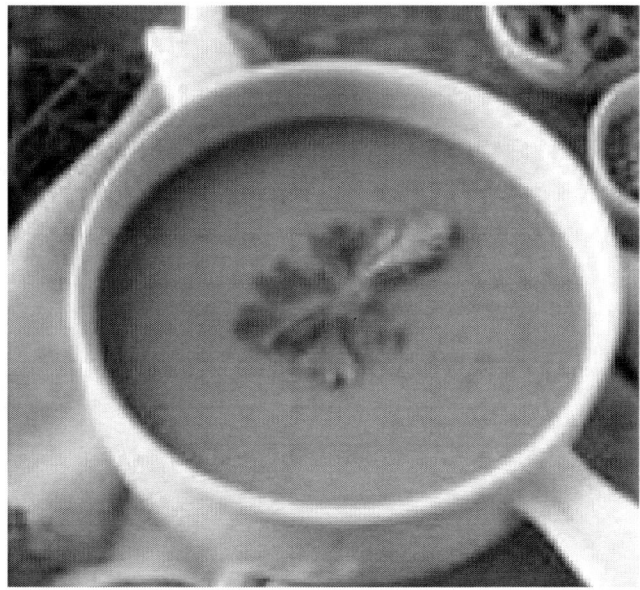

20. Spinach and Potato Stew

Ingredients:
- 1 lb potatoes, peeled and diced
- 4 cups fresh spinach, chopped
- 1 onion, diced
- 2 cloves garlic, minced
- 4 cups low-sodium vegetable broth
- 1 can (14.5 oz) diced tomatoes
- 1 tbsp olive oil
- 1 tsp thyme
- 1/4 tsp paprika

Instructions:
1. In a large pot, heat the olive oil over medium heat. Add the diced onion and minced garlic. Cook until the onion is translucent, about 5 minutes.
2. Add the diced potatoes, vegetable broth, diced tomatoes, thyme, and paprika. Bring to a boil.
3. Reduce the heat and simmer for 20 minutes, or until the potatoes are tender.
4. Stir in the chopped spinach and cook for another 2-3 minutes until wilted.
5. Serve hot.

Nutrition Info (per serving):
- Calories: 180
- Protein: 5g
- Carbohydrates: 32g
- Dietary Fiber: 6g
- Sugars: 7g
- Fat: 4g
- Saturated Fat: 0.5g
- Cholesterol: 0mg
- Sodium: 150mg

Servings: 4
Cooking Time: 30 minutes

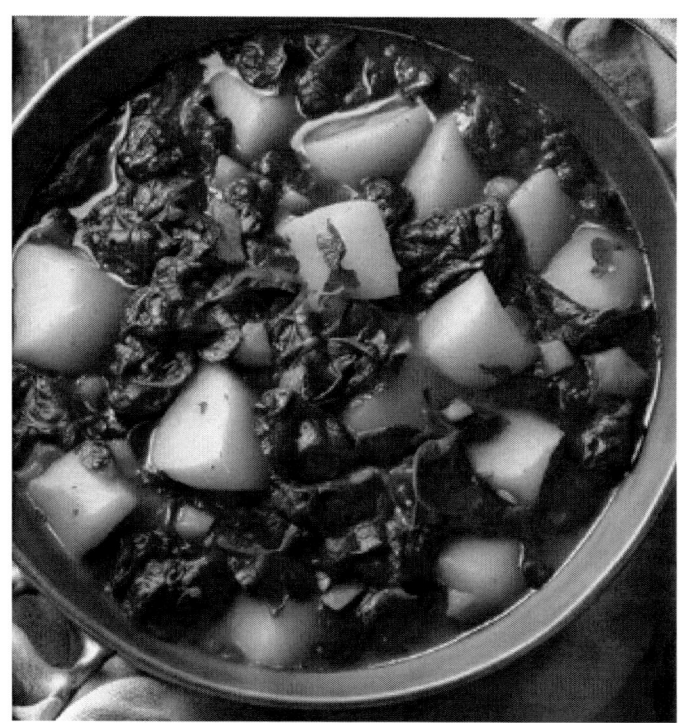

Vegetables

1. Steamed Broccoli with Lemon Zest

Ingredients:
- 1 large head of broccoli, cut into florets
- 1 lemon, zested
- 1 tbsp olive oil
- 1 tbsp lemon juice

Instructions:
1. Fill a large pot with about 1 inch of water and bring to a boil. Place a steamer basket in the pot.
2. Add the broccoli florets to the steamer basket, cover, and steam for about 5-7 minutes, until the broccoli is tender but still bright green.
3. Remove the broccoli from the steamer and place it in a large bowl.
4. Drizzle with olive oil and lemon juice, and sprinkle with lemon zest.
5. Toss gently to combine and serve immediately.

Nutrition Info (per serving):
- Calories: 80
- Protein: 3g
- Carbohydrates: 7g
- Dietary Fiber: 3g
- Sugars: 2g
- Fat: 5g
- Saturated Fat: 1g
- Cholesterol: 0mg
- Sodium: 30mg

Servings: 4
Cooking Time: 10 minutes

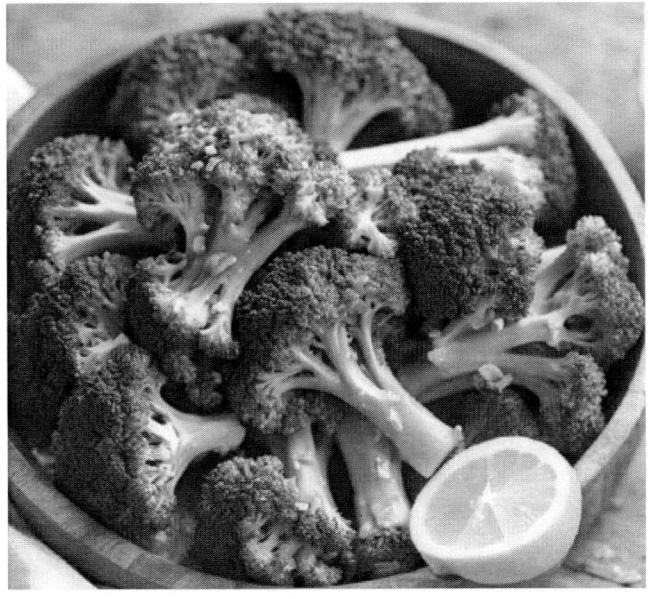

2. Carrot and Zucchini Ribbons

Ingredients:
- 2 large carrots, peeled
- 2 large zucchinis
- 1 tbsp olive oil
- 1 tbsp lemon juice
- 1 tsp fresh thyme, chopped

Instructions:
1. Using a vegetable peeler, create long ribbons from the carrots and zucchinis.
2. In a large skillet, heat the olive oil over medium heat.
3. Add the carrot and zucchini ribbons to the skillet and sauté for 3-4 minutes, until just tender.
4. Remove from heat and toss with lemon juice and fresh thyme.
5. Serve immediately.

Nutrition Info (per serving):
- Calories: 60
- Protein: 1g
- Carbohydrates: 8g
- Dietary Fiber: 2g
- Sugars: 4g
- Fat: 4g
- Saturated Fat: 0.5g
- Cholesterol: 0mg
- Sodium: 10mg

Servings: 4
Cooking Time: 10 minutes

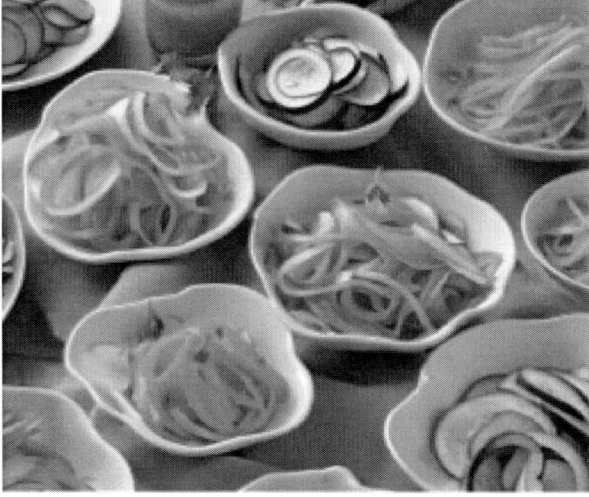

3. Roasted Beetroot with Feta

Ingredients:
- 4 medium beets, peeled and cut into wedges
- 2 tbsp olive oil
- 1/4 cup crumbled feta cheese
- 1 tbsp balsamic vinegar
- 1 tbsp fresh parsley, chopped

Instructions:
1. Preheat your oven to 400°F (200°C). Line a baking sheet with parchment paper.
2. Toss the beet wedges with olive oil and place them on the prepared baking sheet.
3. Roast in the preheated oven for 30-35 minutes, or until the beets are tender.
4. Remove the beets from the oven and transfer to a serving dish.
5. Drizzle with balsamic vinegar and sprinkle with crumbled feta cheese and fresh parsley.
6. Serve warm.

Nutrition Info (per serving):
- Calories: 140
- Protein: 3g
- Carbohydrates: 13g
- Dietary Fiber: 3g
- Sugars: 9g
- Fat: 9g
- Saturated Fat: 3g
- Cholesterol: 10mg
- Sodium: 150mg

Servings: 4
Cooking Time: 40 minutes

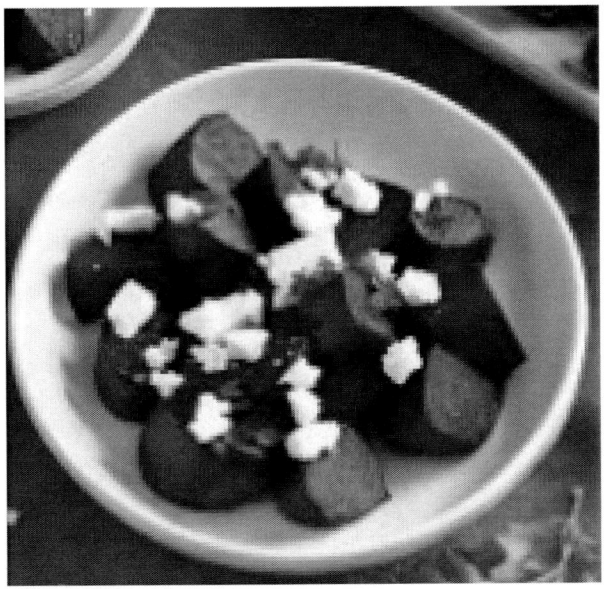

4. Sautéed Green Beans with Almonds
Ingredients:
- 1 lb green beans, trimmed
- 2 tbsp olive oil
- 2 cloves garlic, minced
- 1/4 cup sliced almonds
- 1 tbsp lemon juice

Instructions:
1. Blanch the green beans in a large pot of boiling water for 2-3 minutes until bright green and tender-crisp. Drain and set aside.
2. In a large skillet, heat the olive oil over medium heat.
3. Add the minced garlic and cook for 1-2 minutes until fragrant.
4. Add the blanched green beans and sauté for 3-4 minutes until heated through.
5. Stir in the sliced almonds and cook for another 1-2 minutes until the almonds are lightly toasted.
6. Drizzle with lemon juice and toss to combine.
7. Serve immediately.

Nutrition Info (per serving):
- Calories: 130
- Protein: 3g
- Carbohydrates: 8g
- Dietary Fiber: 4g
- Sugars: 2g
- Fat: 11g
- Saturated Fat: 1g
- Cholesterol: 0mg
- Sodium: 5mg

Servings: 4
Cooking Time: 10 minutes

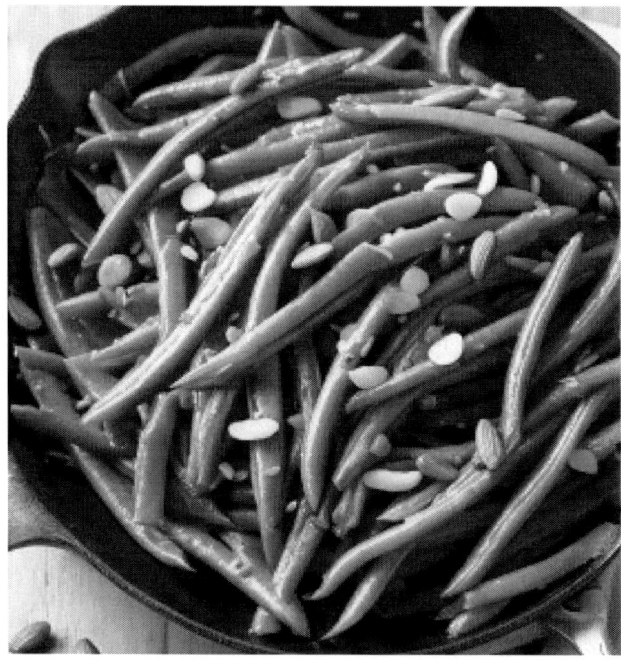

5. Cauliflower Steaks

Ingredients:
- 1 large head of cauliflower
- 2 tbsp olive oil
- 1 tsp paprika
- 1 tsp garlic powder
- 1 tbsp lemon juice
- 1 tbsp fresh parsley, chopped

Instructions:
1. Preheat your oven to 400°F (200°C). Line a baking sheet with parchment paper.
2. Remove the leaves and trim the stem of the cauliflower, leaving the core intact. Slice the cauliflower into 1-inch thick steaks.
3. In a small bowl, mix the olive oil, paprika, and garlic powder.
4. Brush both sides of the cauliflower steaks with the olive oil mixture and place them on the prepared baking sheet.
5. Roast in the preheated oven for 25-30 minutes, flipping halfway through, until the cauliflower is tender and golden brown.
6. Drizzle with lemon juice and sprinkle with fresh parsley before serving.
7. Serve warm.

Nutrition Info (per serving):
- Calories: 90
- Protein: 3g
- Carbohydrates: 8g
- Dietary Fiber: 3g
- Sugars: 3g
- Fat: 7g
- Saturated Fat: 1g
- Cholesterol: 0mg
- Sodium: 25mg

Servings: 4
Cooking Time: 35 minutes

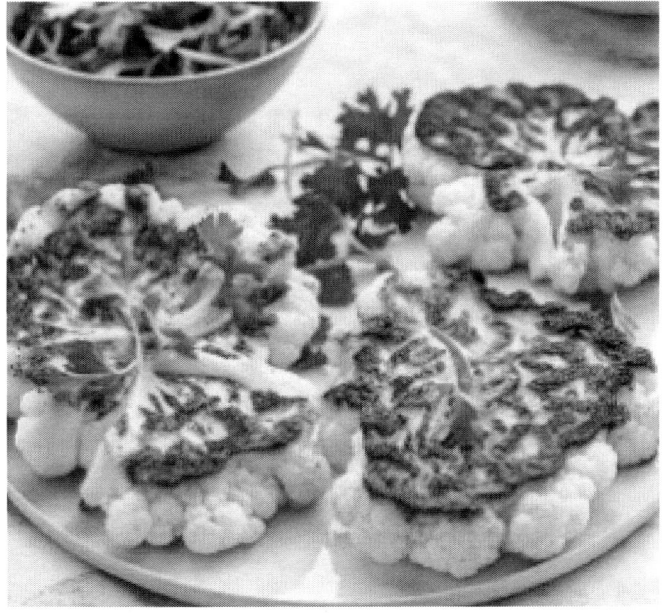

6. Herb Roasted Parsnips

Ingredients:
- 1 lb parsnips, peeled and cut into sticks
- 2 tbsp olive oil
- 1 tsp dried thyme
- 1 tsp dried rosemary
- 1 tbsp fresh parsley, chopped
- 1 tbsp lemon juice

Instructions:
1. Preheat your oven to 400°F (200°C). Line a baking sheet with parchment paper.
2. In a large bowl, toss the parsnips with olive oil, thyme, and rosemary.
3. Spread the parsnips in a single layer on the prepared baking sheet.
4. Roast for 25-30 minutes, or until the parsnips are golden brown and tender, stirring halfway through.
5. Remove from the oven and toss with lemon juice and fresh parsley before serving.
6. Serve warm.

Nutrition Info (per serving):
- Calories: 120
- Protein: 1g
- Carbohydrates: 17g
- Dietary Fiber: 5g
- Sugars: 5g
- Fat: 6g
- Saturated Fat: 1g
- Cholesterol: 0mg
- Sodium: 20mg

Servings: 4

Cooking Time: 35 minutes

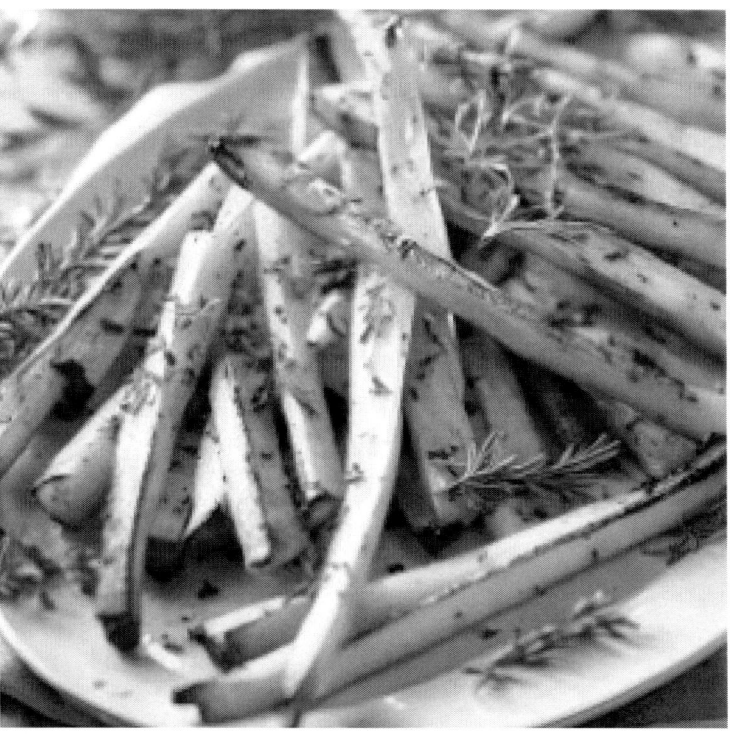

7. Grilled Asparagus with Lemon Butter

Ingredients:
- 1 lb asparagus, trimmed
- 2 tbsp olive oil
- 2 tbsp unsalted butter, melted
- 1 lemon, zested and juiced

Instructions:
1. Preheat your grill to medium-high heat.
2. Toss the asparagus with olive oil until evenly coated.
3. Grill the asparagus for 3-4 minutes on each side, or until tender and slightly charred.
4. In a small bowl, combine the melted butter with lemon zest and lemon juice.
5. Drizzle the lemon butter over the grilled asparagus before serving.
6. Serve warm.

Nutrition Info (per serving):
- Calories: 110
- Protein: 2g
- Carbohydrates: 5g
- Dietary Fiber: 2g
- Sugars: 2g
- Fat: 10g
- Saturated Fat: 4g
- Cholesterol: 10mg
- Sodium: 5mg

Servings: 4
Cooking Time: 10 minutes

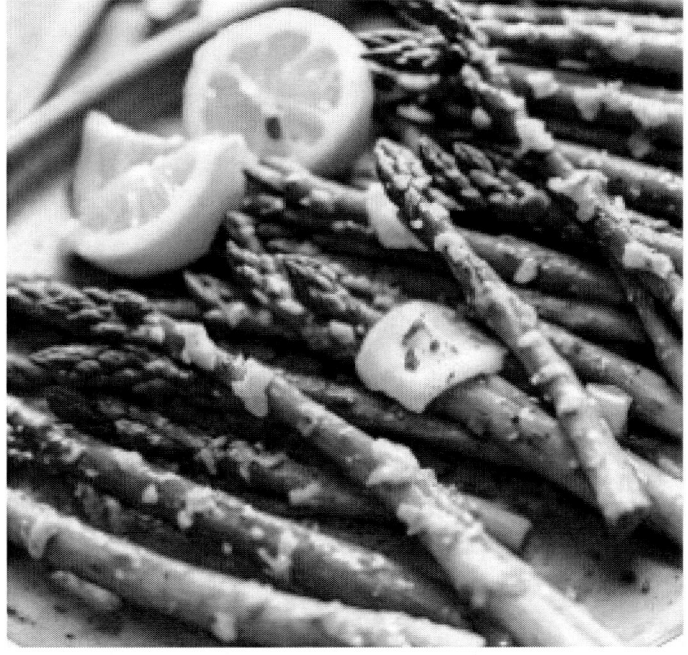

8. Sweet Potato Casserole

Ingredients:
- 4 large sweet potatoes, peeled and cubed
- 1/4 cup unsalted butter, melted
- 1/4 cup honey
- 1/2 cup low-fat milk
- 1 tsp cinnamon
- 1/2 tsp nutmeg
- 1/2 cup chopped pecans

Instructions:
1. Preheat your oven to 350°F (175°C). Grease a 9x13 inch baking dish.
2. Boil the sweet potatoes in a large pot of water until tender, about 15 minutes. Drain and transfer to a large bowl.
3. Mash the sweet potatoes with the melted butter, honey, milk, cinnamon, and nutmeg until smooth.
4. Spread the sweet potato mixture into the prepared baking dish.
5. Sprinkle the chopped pecans evenly over the top.
6. Bake in the preheated oven for 20-25 minutes, or until the casserole is heated through and the pecans are toasted.
7. Serve warm.

Nutrition Info (per serving):
- Calories: 250
- Protein: 3g
- Carbohydrates: 40g
- Dietary Fiber: 6g
- Sugars: 15g
- Fat: 10g
- Saturated Fat: 4g
- Cholesterol: 15mg
- Sodium: 35mg

Servings: 6
Cooking Time: 45 minutes

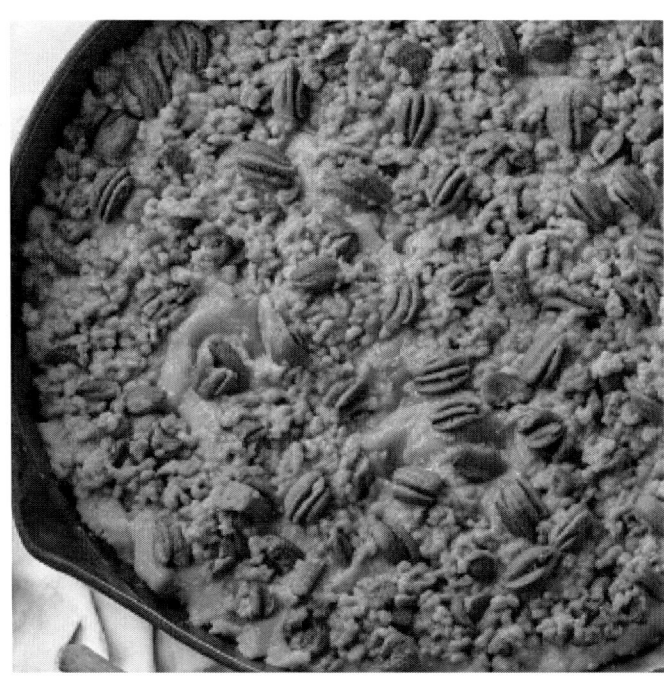

9. Braised Red Cabbage

Ingredients:
- 1 small head of red cabbage, thinly sliced
- 1 apple, peeled and grated
- 1 onion, thinly sliced
- 2 tbsp olive oil
- 1/4 cup apple cider vinegar
- 1/4 cup apple juice
- 1 tbsp brown sugar
- 1/2 tsp ground cloves

Instructions:
1. In a large pot, heat the olive oil over medium heat. Add the sliced onion and cook until softened, about 5 minutes.
2. Add the red cabbage and grated apple to the pot, stirring to combine.
3. Pour in the apple cider vinegar, apple juice, and sprinkle with brown sugar and ground cloves.
4. Bring to a boil, then reduce the heat and simmer, covered, for 30-35 minutes, or until the cabbage is tender.
5. Serve warm.

Nutrition Info (per serving):
- Calories: 100
- Protein: 2g
- Carbohydrates: 18g
- Dietary Fiber: 4g
- Sugars: 12g
- Fat: 3g
- Saturated Fat: 0.5g
- Cholesterol: 0mg
- Sodium: 15mg

Servings: 6
Cooking Time: 40 minutes

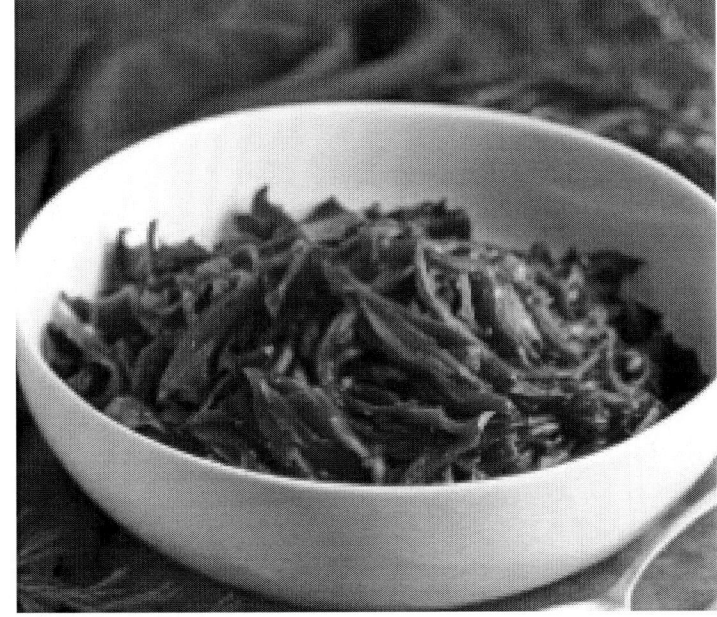

10. Eggplant Parmesan

Ingredients:
- 2 large eggplants, sliced into 1/2-inch rounds
- 1 cup whole wheat bread crumbs
- 1/2 cup grated Parmesan cheese
- 1/2 cup all-purpose flour
- 2 eggs, beaten
- 2 cups marinara sauce
- 1 1/2 cups shredded mozzarella cheese
- 2 tbsp olive oil

Instructions:
1. Preheat your oven to 375°F (190°C). Line a baking sheet with parchment paper.
2. Set up a breading station with three shallow bowls: one with flour, one with beaten eggs, and one with a mixture of bread crumbs and grated Parmesan cheese.
3. Dredge each eggplant slice in the flour, dip in the beaten eggs, and coat with the bread crumb mixture. Place the breaded eggplant slices on the prepared baking sheet.
4. Drizzle the eggplant slices with olive oil and bake for 25-30 minutes, or until golden brown and tender, flipping halfway through.
5. In a 9x13 inch baking dish, spread a thin layer of marinara sauce. Arrange a layer of baked eggplant slices on top. Spoon marinara sauce over the eggplant and sprinkle with shredded mozzarella cheese. Repeat the layers until all ingredients are used, finishing with a layer of marinara sauce and mozzarella cheese.
6. Bake in the preheated oven for 20-25 minutes, or until the cheese is melted and bubbly.
7. Serve warm.

Nutrition Info (per serving):
- Calories: 300
- Protein: 12g
- Carbohydrates: 35g
- Dietary Fiber: 8g
- Sugars: 12g
- Fat: 14g
- Saturated Fat: 6g
- Cholesterol: 75mg
- Sodium: 350mg

Servings: 6
Cooking Time: 1 hour

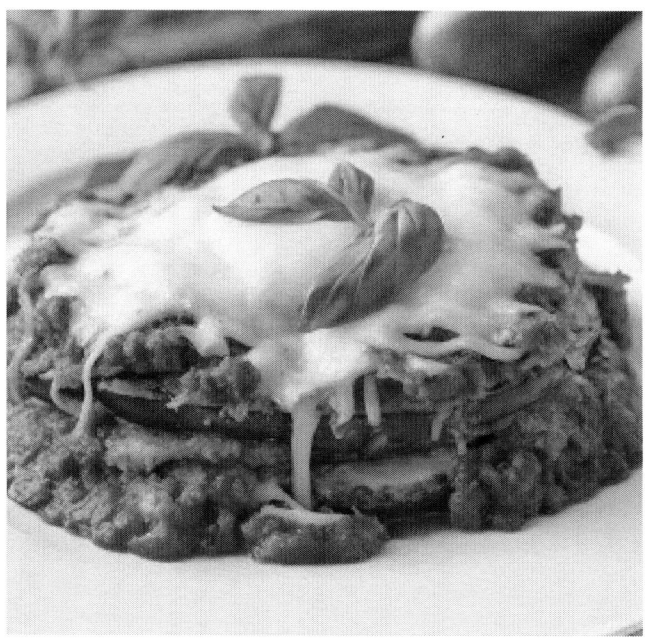

11. Roasted Brussels Sprouts with Garlic

Ingredients:
- 1 lb Brussels sprouts, trimmed and halved
- 3 cloves garlic, minced
- 2 tbsp olive oil
- 1 tbsp balsamic vinegar

Instructions:
1. Preheat your oven to 400°F (200°C). Line a baking sheet with parchment paper.
2. In a large bowl, toss the Brussels sprouts with olive oil and minced garlic.
3. Spread the Brussels sprouts in a single layer on the prepared baking sheet.
4. Roast for 20-25 minutes, stirring halfway through, until the Brussels sprouts are golden brown and tender.
5. Remove from the oven and drizzle with balsamic vinegar before serving.
6. Serve warm.

Nutrition Info (per serving):
- Calories: 110
- Protein: 3g
- Carbohydrates: 11g
- Dietary Fiber: 4g
- Sugars: 3g
- Fat: 7g
- Saturated Fat: 1g
- Cholesterol: 0mg
- Sodium: 20mg

Servings: 4
Cooking Time: 30 minutes

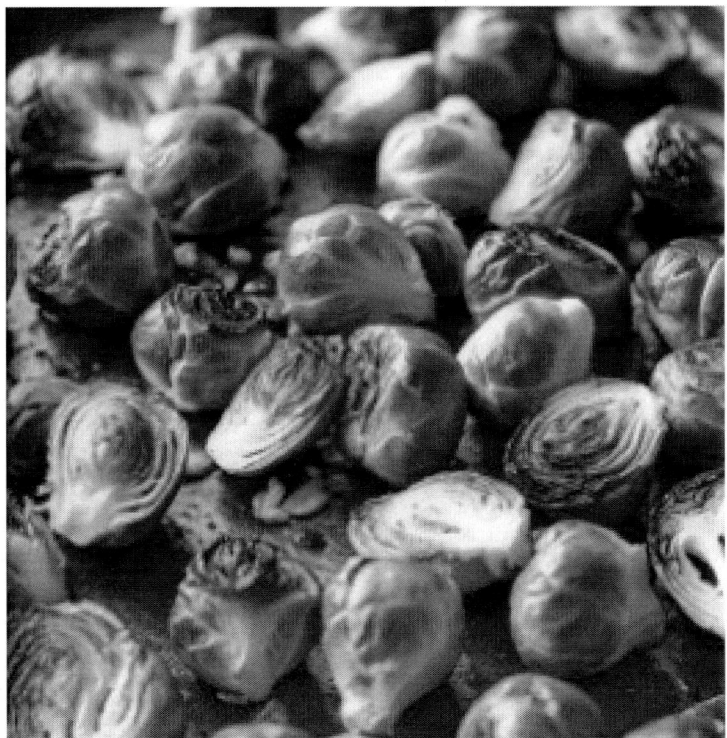

12. Bok Choy with Oyster Sauce

Ingredients:
- 1 lb baby bok choy, halved lengthwise
- 2 tbsp olive oil
- 3 cloves garlic, minced
- 2 tbsp oyster sauce
- 1 tbsp low-sodium soy sauce
- 1 tsp sesame oil

Instructions:
1. In a large skillet, heat the olive oil over medium heat. Add the minced garlic and cook for 1-2 minutes until fragrant.
2. Add the bok choy, cut side down, and cook for 3-4 minutes until slightly browned.
3. Flip the bok choy and add the oyster sauce, soy sauce, and sesame oil. Cook for another 2-3 minutes until the bok choy is tender and the sauce is heated through.
4. Serve immediately.

Nutrition Info (per serving):
- Calories: 90
- Protein: 3g
- Carbohydrates: 6g
- Dietary Fiber: 2g
- Sugars: 2g
- Fat: 7g
- Saturated Fat: 1g
- Cholesterol: 0mg
- Sodium: 220mg

Servings: 4
Cooking Time: 10 minutes

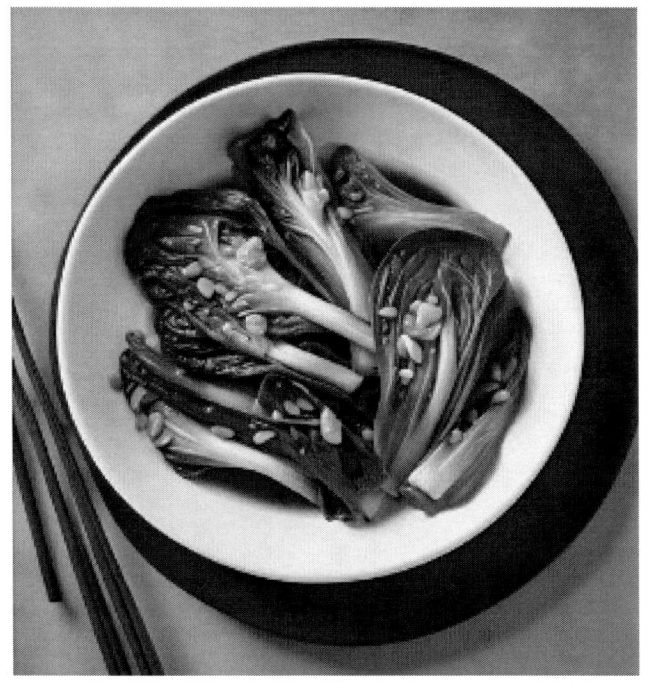

13. Corn on the Cob with Herb Butter

Ingredients:
- 4 ears of corn, husked
- 4 tbsp unsalted butter, softened
- 1 tbsp fresh parsley, chopped
- 1 tsp fresh thyme, chopped
- 1 tsp lemon zest

Instructions:
1. Bring a large pot of water to a boil. Add the corn and cook for 5-7 minutes until tender.
2. In a small bowl, mix the softened butter with chopped parsley, thyme, and lemon zest.
3. Drain the corn and spread the herb butter evenly over each ear.
4. Serve immediately.

Nutrition Info (per serving):
- Calories: 170
- Protein: 3g
- Carbohydrates: 19g
- Dietary Fiber: 2g
- Sugars: 5g
- Fat: 10g
- Saturated Fat: 6g
- Cholesterol: 25mg
- Sodium: 30mg

Servings: 4
Cooking Time: 10 minutes

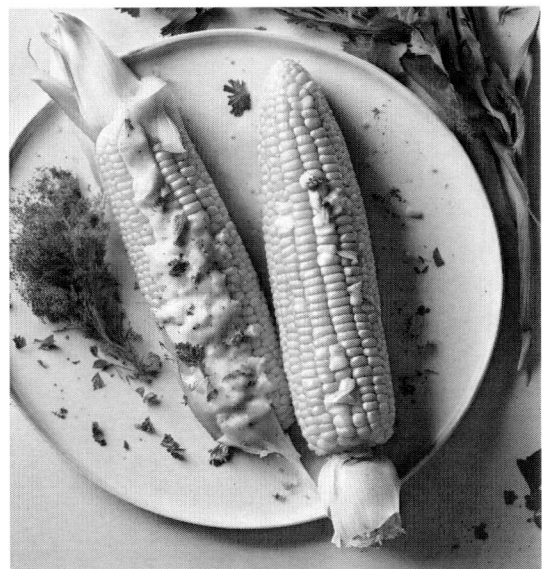

14. Cucumber Salad with Dill

Ingredients:
- 2 large cucumbers, thinly sliced
- 1/4 cup red onion, thinly sliced
- 3 tbsp white vinegar
- 2 tbsp olive oil
- 1 tbsp fresh dill, chopped
- 1 tsp honey

Instructions:
1. In a large bowl, combine the sliced cucumbers and red onion.
2. In a small bowl, whisk together the white vinegar, olive oil, chopped dill, and honey.
3. Pour the dressing over the cucumbers and onion, and toss to combine.
4. Chill in the refrigerator for at least 30 minutes before serving.
5. Serve cold.

Nutrition Info (per serving):
- Calories: 70
- Protein: 1g
- Carbohydrates: 6g
- Dietary Fiber: 1g
- Sugars: 4g
- Fat: 5g
- Saturated Fat: 1g
- Cholesterol: 0mg
- Sodium: 5mg

Servings: 4

Cooking Time: 10 minutes + 30 minutes chilling

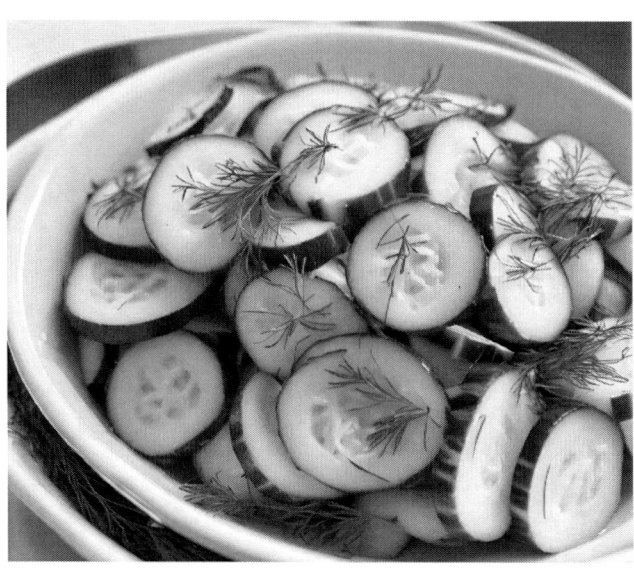

15. Spaghetti Squash with Tomato Sauce

Ingredients:
- 1 large spaghetti squash
- 2 tbsp olive oil
- 1 onion, diced
- 2 cloves garlic, minced
- 1 can (14.5 oz) diced tomatoes
- 1 tbsp tomato paste
- 1 tsp dried basil
- 1 tsp dried oregano
- 1/4 cup grated Parmesan cheese (optional)

Instructions:
1. Preheat your oven to 375°F (190°C). Line a baking sheet with parchment paper.
2. Cut the spaghetti squash in half lengthwise and scoop out the seeds. Drizzle the insides with 1 tbsp olive oil.
3. Place the squash halves cut side down on the prepared baking sheet. Roast for 35-40 minutes, or until the squash is tender and can be easily shredded with a fork.
4. While the squash is roasting, heat the remaining 1 tbsp olive oil in a large skillet over medium heat. Add the diced onion and minced garlic, and cook until the onion is translucent, about 5 minutes.
5. Stir in the diced tomatoes, tomato paste, basil, and oregano. Simmer for 10-15 minutes, stirring occasionally.
6. Once the squash is done, use a fork to shred the flesh into spaghetti-like strands.
7. Serve the spaghetti squash topped with the tomato sauce and grated Parmesan cheese, if desired.

Nutrition Info (per serving):
- Calories: 140
- Protein: 3g
- Carbohydrates: 18g
- Dietary Fiber: 4g
- Sugars: 8g
- Fat: 7g
- Saturated Fat: 1g
- Cholesterol: 0mg
- Sodium: 150mg

Servings: 4
Cooking Time: 50 minutes

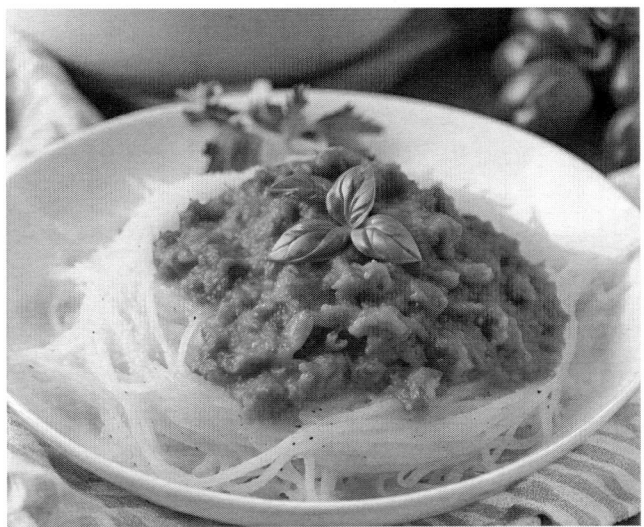

16. Roasted Garlic Mashed Potatoes

Ingredients:
- 4 large potatoes, peeled and cubed
- 1 whole garlic bulb
- 2 tbsp olive oil
- 1/2 cup low-fat milk
- 2 tbsp unsalted butter
- 1 tbsp fresh parsley, chopped

Instructions:
1. Preheat your oven to 400°F (200°C). Cut the top off the garlic bulb to expose the cloves. Drizzle with 1 tbsp olive oil, wrap in foil, and roast for 30-35 minutes until soft.
2. Boil the cubed potatoes in a large pot of water until tender, about 15-20 minutes. Drain and return to the pot.
3. Squeeze the roasted garlic cloves out of their skins and add to the potatoes.
4. Add the remaining 1 tbsp olive oil, low-fat milk, and unsalted butter to the potatoes. Mash until smooth.
5. Stir in the chopped parsley.
6. Serve warm.

Nutrition Info (per serving):
- Calories: 180
- Protein: 3g
- Carbohydrates: 30g
- Dietary Fiber: 4g
- Sugars: 2g
- Fat: 7g
- Saturated Fat: 3g
- Cholesterol: 10mg
- Sodium: 30mg

Servings: 4
Cooking Time: 45 minutes

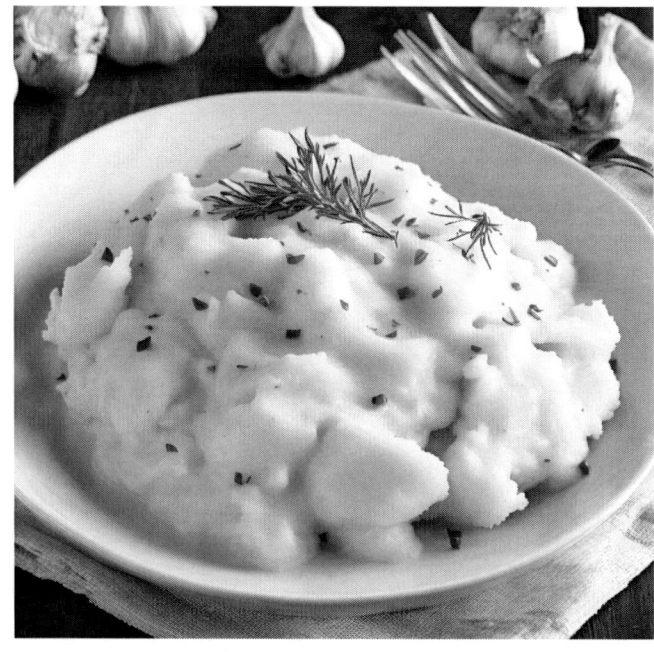

17. Pea and Mint Puree

Ingredients:
- 2 cups frozen peas
- 1/4 cup fresh mint leaves
- 1 tbsp olive oil
- 1/4 cup low-fat Greek yogurt

Instructions:
1. Cook the frozen peas in a pot of boiling water for 3-4 minutes until tender. Drain.
2. In a food processor, combine the cooked peas, fresh mint leaves, olive oil, and Greek yogurt. Blend until smooth.
3. Serve warm or chilled.

Nutrition Info (per serving):
- Calories: 100
- Protein: 4g
- Carbohydrates: 14g
- Dietary Fiber: 4g
- Sugars: 5g
- Fat: 4g
- Saturated Fat: 1g
- Cholesterol: 0mg
- Sodium: 40mg

Servings: 4
Cooking Time: 10 minutes

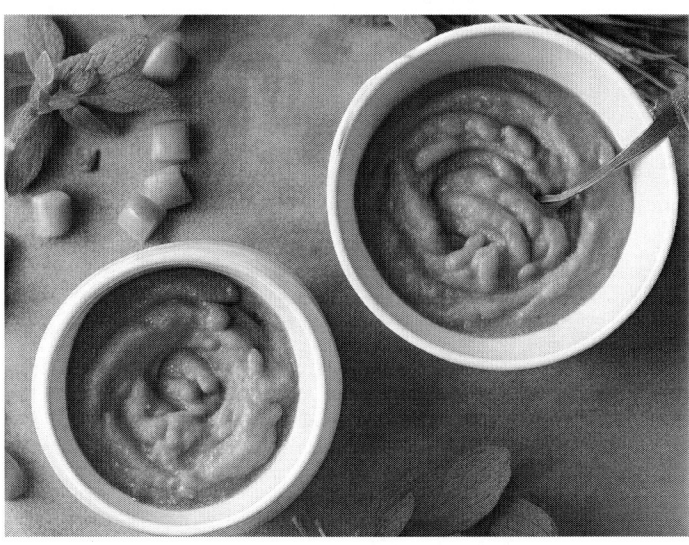

18. Roasted Turnips with Rosemary

Ingredients:
- 1 lb turnips, peeled and cut into wedges
- 2 tbsp olive oil
- 1 tsp dried rosemary
- 1 tbsp balsamic vinegar

Instructions:
1. Preheat your oven to 400°F (200°C). Line a baking sheet with parchment paper.
2. In a large bowl, toss the turnip wedges with olive oil and dried rosemary.
3. Spread the turnips in a single layer on the prepared baking sheet.
4. Roast for 25-30 minutes, or until the turnips are golden brown and tender, stirring halfway through.
5. Remove from the oven and drizzle with balsamic vinegar before serving.
6. Serve warm.

Nutrition Info (per serving):
- Calories: 100
- Protein: 1g
- Carbohydrates: 12g
- Dietary Fiber: 3g
- Sugars: 5g
- Fat: 6g
- Saturated Fat: 1g
- Cholesterol: 0mg
- Sodium: 25mg

Servings: 4
Cooking Time: 35 minutes

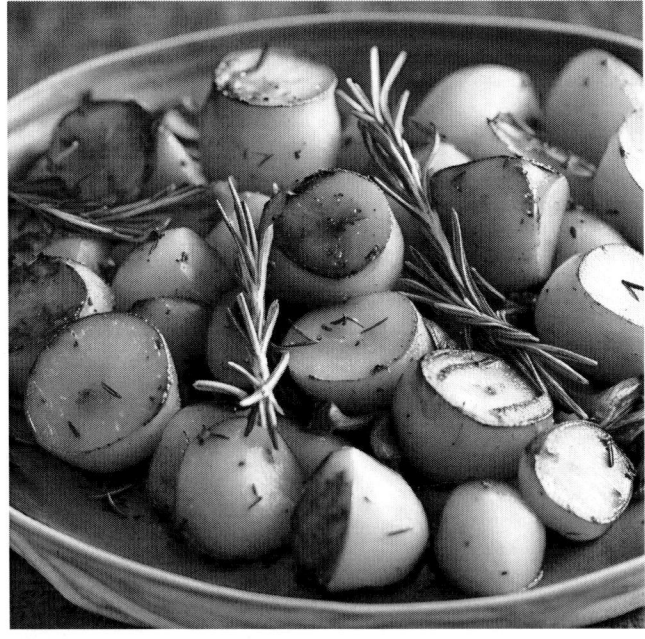

19. Swiss Chard with Pine Nuts

Ingredients:
- 1 bunch Swiss chard, stems removed and leaves chopped
- 2 tbsp olive oil
- 2 cloves garlic, minced
- 1/4 cup pine nuts
- 1 tbsp lemon juice

Instructions:
1. In a large skillet, heat the olive oil over medium heat. Add the minced garlic and cook for 1-2 minutes until fragrant.
2. Add the chopped Swiss chard to the skillet and sauté for 5-7 minutes until wilted.
3. Stir in the pine nuts and cook for another 2-3 minutes until the pine nuts are lightly toasted.
4. Drizzle with lemon juice before serving.
5. Serve warm.

Nutrition Info (per serving):
- Calories: 130
- Protein: 3g
- Carbohydrates: 7g
- Dietary Fiber: 3g
- Sugars: 1g
- Fat: 11g
- Saturated Fat: 1.5g
- Cholesterol: 0mg
- Sodium: 40mg

Servings: 4
Cooking Time: 10 minutes

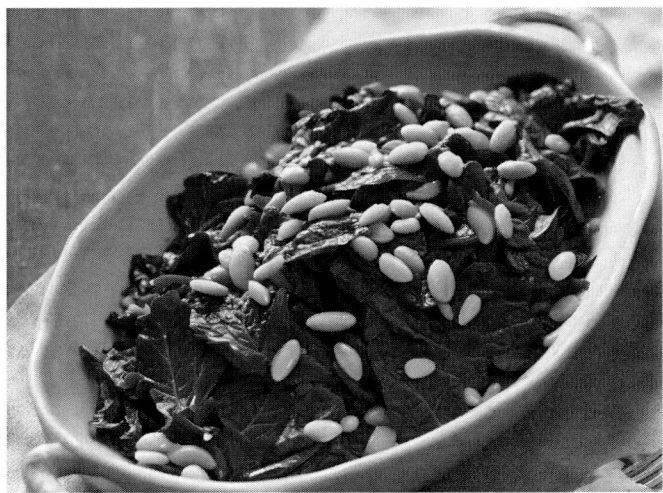

20. Fennel and Orange Salad

Ingredients:
- 2 large fennel bulbs, thinly sliced
- 2 large oranges, peeled and segmented
- 1/4 cup red onion, thinly sliced
- 2 tbsp olive oil
- 1 tbsp white wine vinegar
- 1 tbsp fresh mint, chopped

Instructions:
1. In a large bowl, combine the thinly sliced fennel, orange segments, and red onion.
2. In a small bowl, whisk together the olive oil and white wine vinegar.
3. Pour the dressing over the fennel and oranges, and toss gently to combine.
4. Sprinkle with fresh mint before serving.
5. Serve chilled.

Nutrition Info (per serving):
- Calories: 110
- Protein: 2g
- Carbohydrates: 17g
- Dietary Fiber: 5g
- Sugars: 10g
- Fat: 5g
- Saturated Fat: 1g
- Cholesterol: 0mg
- Sodium: 20mg

Servings: 4
Cooking Time: 15 minutes

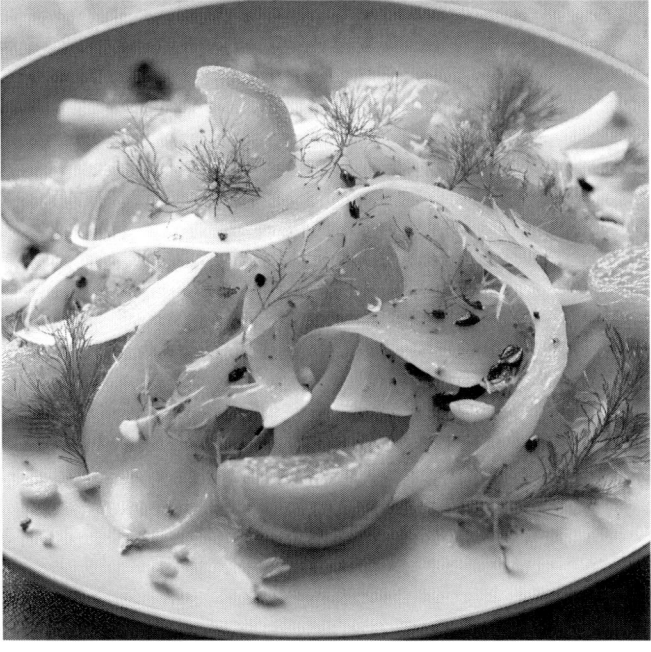

10-WEEK MEAL PLAN.

Week 1
Monday:
- Breakfast: Almond Butter Banana Smoothie
- Lunch: Chicken Salad with Greek Yogurt Dressing
- Dinner: Ginger Salmon Stir-Fry

Tuesday:
- Breakfast: Savory Porridge with Egg
- Lunch: Zucchini Basil Soup
- Dinner: Roasted Beetroot with Feta

Wednesday:
- Breakfast: Granola and Fruit Medley
- Lunch: Carrot and Zucchini Ribbons
- Dinner: Spaghetti Squash with Tomato Sauce

Thursday:
- Breakfast: Gluten-Free Blueberry Waffles
- Lunch: Lentil and Carrot Soup
- Dinner: Turkey Sweet Potato Skillet

Friday:
- Breakfast: Tofu Scramble with Avocado
- Lunch: Pea and Mint Puree
- Dinner: Baked Cod with Lemon and Dill

Saturday:
- Breakfast: Sweet Corn Porridge
- Lunch: Roasted Turnips with Rosemary
- Dinner: Moroccan Lentil Soup

Sunday:
- Breakfast: Overnight Barley
- Lunch: Roasted Brussels Sprouts with Garlic
- Dinner: Simple Grilled Tilapia

Week 2
Monday:
- Breakfast: Protein-Packed French Toast
- Lunch: Broccoli and Cheese Soup
- Dinner: Chicken and Broccoli Alfredo

Tuesday:
- Breakfast: Spinach and Cheese Stuffed Mushrooms
- Lunch: Braised Red Cabbage
- Dinner: Sea Bass with Roasted Vegetables

Wednesday:
- Breakfast: Veggie-Packed Breakfast Burritos
- Lunch: Swiss Chard with Pine Nuts
- Dinner: Split Pea and Ham Soup

Thursday:
- Breakfast: Baked Sweet Potato with Yogurt
- Lunch: Fennel and Orange Salad
- Dinner: Italian Wedding Soup

Friday:
- Breakfast: Sweet Corn Porridge
- Lunch: Shrimp and Avocado Salad
- Dinner: Cauliflower Steaks

Saturday:
- Breakfast: Overnight Barley
- Lunch: Corn on the Cob with Herb Butter
- Dinner: Thai Coconut Chicken Soup

Sunday:
- Breakfast: Zucchini Bread
- Lunch: Steamed Broccoli with Lemon Zest
- Dinner: Vegetable Beef Soup

Week 3

Monday:
- Breakfast: Turkey and Spinach Mini Quiches
- Lunch: Sweet Potato Casserole
- Dinner: Parmesan Crusted Halibut

Tuesday:
- Breakfast: Pumpkin Pancakes
- Lunch: Bok Choy with Oyster Sauce
- Dinner: Moroccan Spiced Chicken Stew

Wednesday:
- Breakfast: Berry Yogurt Parfait
- Lunch: Kale and White Bean Soup
- Dinner: Clam Soup with Vegetables

Thursday:
- Breakfast: Banana Almond Muffins
- Lunch: Cucumber Salad with Dill
- Dinner: Crab and Spinach Stuffed Mushrooms

Friday:
- Breakfast: Savory Muffins
- Lunch: Spinach and Potato Stew
- Dinner: Poached Haddock in Milk

Saturday:
- Breakfast: Lentil and Veggie Breakfast Salad
- Lunch: Asparagus Soup
- Dinner: Turkey Quinoa Stuffed Peppers

Sunday:
- Breakfast: Savory Porridge with Egg
- Lunch: Carrot and Zucchini Ribbons
- Dinner: Mild White Fish Soup

Week 4

Monday:
- Breakfast: Granola and Fruit Medley
- Lunch: Chicken Ginger Noodle Soup
- Dinner: Roasted Beetroot with Feta

Tuesday:
- Breakfast: Gluten-Free Blueberry Waffles
- Lunch: Turkey Breast with Sweet Potato Mash
- Dinner: Fish Fillet with Light Dill Sauce

Wednesday:
- Breakfast: Tofu Scramble with Avocado
- Lunch: Roasted Turnips with Rosemary
- Dinner: Shrimp and Spinach Quiche

Thursday:
- Breakfast: Sweet Corn Porridge
- Lunch: Broccoli and Cheese Soup
- Dinner: Baked Turkey Meatballs with Spinach

Friday:
- Breakfast: Overnight Barley
- Lunch: Roasted Brussels Sprouts with Garlic
- Dinner: Lemon Herb Roasted Chicken

Saturday:
- Breakfast: Zucchini Bread
- Lunch: Steamed Broccoli with Lemon Zest
- Dinner: Chicken Paillard with Steamed Greens

Sunday:
- Breakfast: Protein-Packed French Toast
- Lunch: Pea and Mint Puree
- Dinner: Roasted Garlic Mashed Potatoes

Week 5

Monday:
- Breakfast: Spinach and Cheese Stuffed Mushrooms
- Lunch: Split Pea and Ham Soup
- Dinner: Tuna Steak with Tomato Salsa

Tuesday:
- Breakfast: Veggie-Packed Breakfast Burritos
- Lunch: Bok Choy with Oyster Sauce
- Dinner: Grilled Salmon with Mango Salsa

Wednesday:
- Breakfast: Baked Sweet Potato with Yogurt
- Lunch: Sweet Potato Casserole
- Dinner: Chicken Stew with Soft Vegetables

Thursday:
- Breakfast: Sweet Corn Porridge
- Lunch: Carrot and Zucchini Ribbons
- Dinner: Mulligatawny Soup

Friday:
- Breakfast: Overnight Barley
- Lunch: Swiss Chard with Pine Nuts
- Dinner: Mackerel Pate

Saturday:
- Breakfast: Zucchini Bread
- Lunch: Corn on the Cob with Herb Butter
- Dinner: Chicken and Broccoli Alfredo

Sunday:
- Breakfast: Savory Muffins
- Lunch: Spinach and Potato Stew
- Dinner: Oxtail Stew

Week 6

Monday:
- Breakfast: Almond Butter Banana Smoothie
- Lunch: Creamy Chicken and Mushroom Soup
- Dinner: Grilled Asparagus with Lemon Butter

Tuesday:
- Breakfast: Savory Porridge with Egg
- Lunch: Sweet Potato Casserole
- Dinner: Baked Tilapia with Oats Crust

Wednesday:
- Breakfast: Granola and Fruit Medley
- Lunch: Turkey and Zucchini Burgers
- Dinner: Clam Soup with Vegetables

Thursday:
- Breakfast: Gluten-Free Blueberry Waffles
- Lunch: Carrot and Zucchini Ribbons
- Dinner: Simple Poached Chicken

Friday:
- Breakfast: Tofu Scramble with Avocado
- Lunch: Cucumber Salad with Dill
- Dinner: Crab and Spinach Stuffed Mushrooms

Saturday:
- Breakfast: Sweet Corn Porridge
- Lunch: Lentil and Carrot Soup
- Dinner: Baked Cod with Lemon and Dill

Sunday:
- Breakfast: Overnight Barley
- Lunch: Roasted Brussels Sprouts with Garlic
- Dinner: Moroccan Spiced Chicken Stew

Week 7

Monday:
- Breakfast: Protein-Packed French Toast
- Lunch: Shrimp and Avocado Salad
- Dinner: Parmesan Crusted Halibut

Tuesday:
- Breakfast: Spinach and Cheese Stuffed Mushrooms
- Lunch: Roasted Turnips with Rosemary
- Dinner: Thai Coconut Chicken Soup

Wednesday:
- Breakfast: Veggie-Packed Breakfast Burritos
- Lunch: Swiss Chard with Pine Nuts
- Dinner: Sea Bass with Roasted Vegetables

Thursday:
- Breakfast: Baked Sweet Potato with Yogurt
- Lunch: Pea and Mint Puree
- Dinner: Italian Wedding Soup

Friday:
- Breakfast: Sweet Corn Porridge
- Lunch: Steamed Broccoli with Lemon Zest
- Dinner: Vegetable Beef Soup

Saturday:
- Breakfast: Overnight Barley
- Lunch: Broccoli and Cheese Soup
- Dinner: Chicken Paillard with Steamed Greens

Sunday:
- Breakfast: Zucchini Bread
- Lunch: Fennel and Orange Salad
- Dinner: Fish Fillet with Light Dill Sauce

Week 8

Monday:
- Breakfast: Turkey and Spinach Mini Quiches
- Lunch: Corn on the Cob with Herb Butter
- Dinner: Shrimp and Spinach Quiche

Tuesday:
- Breakfast: Pumpkin Pancakes
- Lunch: Braised Red Cabbage
- Dinner: Baked Turkey Meatballs with Spinach

Wednesday:
- Breakfast: Berry Yogurt Parfait
- Lunch: Carrot and Zucchini Ribbons
- Dinner: Split Pea and Ham Soup

Thursday:
- Breakfast: Banana Almond Muffins
- Lunch: Spinach and Potato Stew
- Dinner: Oxtail Stew

Friday:
- Breakfast: Savory Muffins
- Lunch: Cucumber Salad with Dill
- Dinner: Grilled Salmon with Mango Salsa

Saturday:
- Breakfast: Lentil and Veggie Breakfast Salad
- Lunch: Broccoli and Cheese Soup
- Dinner: Baked Tilapia with Oats Crust

Sunday:
- Breakfast: Savory Porridge with Egg
- Lunch: Sweet Potato Casserole
- Dinner: Poached Haddock in Milk

Week 9

Monday:
- Breakfast: Granola and Fruit Medley
- Lunch: Kale and White Bean Soup
- Dinner: Chicken Stew with Soft Vegetables

Tuesday:
- Breakfast: Gluten-Free Blueberry Waffles
- Lunch: Roasted Turnips with Rosemary
- Dinner: Mild White Fish Soup

Wednesday:
- Breakfast: Tofu Scramble with Avocado
- Lunch: Swiss Chard with Pine Nuts
- Dinner: Fish Fillet with Light Dill Sauce

Thursday:
- Breakfast: Sweet Corn Porridge
- Lunch: Pea and Mint Puree
- Dinner: Chicken Ginger Noodle Soup

Friday:
- Breakfast: Overnight Barley
- Lunch: Steamed Broccoli with Lemon Zest
- Dinner: Moroccan Lentil Soup

Saturday:
- Breakfast: Zucchini Bread
- Lunch: Corn on the Cob with Herb Butter
- Dinner: Sea Bass with Roasted Vegetables

Sunday:
- Breakfast: Protein-Packed French Toast
- Lunch: Fennel and Orange Salad
- Dinner: Vegetable Beef Soup

Week 10

Monday:
- Breakfast: Spinach and Cheese Stuffed Mushrooms
- Lunch: Lentil and Carrot Soup
- Dinner: Baked Cod with Lemon and Dill

Tuesday:
- Breakfast: Veggie-Packed Breakfast Burritos
- Lunch: Braised Red Cabbage
- Dinner: Moroccan Spiced Chicken Stew

Wednesday:
- Breakfast: Baked Sweet Potato with Yogurt
- Lunch: Roasted Brussels Sprouts with Garlic
- Dinner: Chicken Paillard with Steamed Greens

Thursday:
- Breakfast: Sweet Corn Porridge
- Lunch: Cucumber Salad with Dill
- Dinner: Parmesan Crusted Halibut

Friday:
- Breakfast: Overnight Barley
- Lunch: Carrot and Zucchini Ribbons
- Dinner: Split Pea and Ham Soup

Saturday:
- Breakfast: Zucchini Bread
- Lunch: Pea and Mint Puree
- Dinner: Thai Coconut Chicken Soup

Sunday:
- Breakfast: Savory Muffins
- Lunch: Swiss Chard with Pine Nuts
- Dinner: Simple Poached Chicken

WEEKLY MEAL PLANNER + WORKBOOK

	BREAKFAST	LUNCH	DINNER	SNACKS
MONDAY				
TUESDAY				
WEDNESDAY				
THURSDAY				
FRIDAY				
SATURDAY				
SUNDAY				

Describe your typical daily routine before undergoing chemotherapy. How did your eating habits fit into this routine?

....

....

....

....

....

....

WEEKLY MEAL PLANNER + WORKBOOK

	BREAKFAST	LUNCH	DINNER	SNACKS
MONDAY				
TUESDAY				
WEDNESDAY				
THURSDAY				
FRIDAY				
SATURDAY				
SUNDAY				

What were your favorite foods or meals before starting chemotherapy? How have your preferences changed since then?

....

....

....

....

....

....

WEEKLY MEAL PLANNER + WORKBOOK

	BREAKFAST	LUNCH	DINNER	SNACKS
MONDAY				
TUESDAY				
WEDNESDAY				
THURSDAY				
FRIDAY				
SATURDAY				
SUNDAY				

How did you typically manage stress or emotions before chemotherapy? Has this changed during treatment?

....

....

....

....

....

....

WEEKLY MEAL PLANNER + WORKBOOK

	BREAKFAST	LUNCH	DINNER	SNACKS
MONDAY				
TUESDAY				
WEDNESDAY				
THURSDAY				
FRIDAY				
SATURDAY				
SUNDAY				

Consider your social life before chemotherapy. How did meals and gatherings with friends or family influence your eating habits?

....

....

....

....

....

....

WEEKLY MEAL PLANNER + WORKBOOK

	BREAKFAST	LUNCH	DINNER	SNACKS
MONDAY				
TUESDAY				
WEDNESDAY				
THURSDAY				
FRIDAY				
SATURDAY				
SUNDAY				

List three foods or beverages you consumed regularly before chemotherapy that may need to be adjusted or avoided on a chemo diet. Why are these adjustments necessary?

....

....

....

....

....

....

WEEKLY MEAL PLANNER + WORKBOOK

	BREAKFAST	LUNCH	DINNER	SNACKS
MONDAY				
TUESDAY				
WEDNESDAY				
THURSDAY				
FRIDAY				
SATURDAY				
SUNDAY				

What were your main sources of hydration before chemotherapy, and how do you plan to maintain adequate hydration during treatment?

....

....

....

....

....

....

WEEKLY MEAL PLANNER + WORKBOOK

	BREAKFAST	LUNCH	DINNER	SNACKS
MONDAY				
TUESDAY				
WEDNESDAY				
THURSDAY				
FRIDAY				
SATURDAY				
SUNDAY				

Think about your cooking skills before chemotherapy. What new cooking techniques or recipes are you interested in trying to support your dietary needs now?

....

....

....

....

....

....

WEEKLY MEAL PLANNER + WORKBOOK

	BREAKFAST	LUNCH	DINNER	SNACKS
MONDAY				
TUESDAY				
WEDNESDAY				
THURSDAY				
FRIDAY				
SATURDAY				
SUNDAY				

What are your main concerns or challenges about starting a chemo diet? How do you plan to address them?

....

....

....

....

....

....

WEEKLY MEAL PLANNER + WORKBOOK

	BREAKFAST	LUNCH	DINNER	SNACKS
MONDAY				
TUESDAY				
WEDNESDAY				
THURSDAY				
FRIDAY				
SATURDAY				
SUNDAY				

Identify three new foods or ingredients you're willing to incorporate into your diet to support your recovery. What benefits do you expect from including these items?

....

....

....

....

....

....

WEEKLY MEAL PLANNER + WORKBOOK

	BREAKFAST	LUNCH	DINNER	SNACKS
MONDAY				
TUESDAY				
WEDNESDAY				
THURSDAY				
FRIDAY				
SATURDAY				
SUNDAY				

Consider your support system. How can family and friends assist you in maintaining a chemo diet and overall wellness during treatment?

....

....

....

....

....

....

WEEKLY MEAL PLANNER + WORKBOOK

	BREAKFAST	LUNCH	DINNER	SNACKS
MONDAY				
TUESDAY				
WEDNESDAY				
THURSDAY				
FRIDAY				
SATURDAY				
SUNDAY				

Reflect on any changes in appetite or taste preferences since starting chemotherapy. How will you adapt your meals to accommodate these changes?

....

....

....

....

....

....

WEEKLY MEAL PLANNER + WORKBOOK

	BREAKFAST	LUNCH	DINNER	SNACKS
MONDAY				
TUESDAY				
WEDNESDAY				
THURSDAY				
FRIDAY				
SATURDAY				
SUNDAY				

Reflect on your goals for following a chemo diet. How will you measure success and adjust your approach based on your progress and experiences?

....

....

....

....

....

....

Scan the QR code below to get a surprise bonus!

Manufactured by Amazon.ca
Acheson, AB

15494389R00085